TREATMENT OF
STRESS RESPONSE
SYNDROMES

TREATMENT OF STRESS RESPONSE SYNDROMES

Mardi J. Horowitz, M.D.

Professor of Psychiatry
University of California, San Francisco

American
Psychiatric
Publishing, Inc.

Washington, DC
London, England

Note: The authors have worked to ensure that all information in this book is accurate at the time of publication and consistent with general psychiatric and medical standards, and that information concerning drug dosages, schedules, and routes of administration is accurate at the time of publication and consistent with standards set by the U. S. Food and Drug Administration and the general medical community. As medical research and practice continue to advance, however, therapeutic standards may change. Moreover, specific situations may require a specific therapeutic response not included in this book. For these reasons and because human and mechanical errors sometimes occur, we recommend that readers follow the advice of physicians directly involved in their care or the care of a member of their family.

Typeset in Adobe's Janson Text and DINNeuzeitGrotesk.

Copyright © 2003 American Psychiatric Publishing, Inc.
ALL RIGHTS RESERVED

Manufactured in Canada on acid-free paper
07   06   05   04   03   5   4   3   2   1
First Edition

American Psychiatric Publishing, Inc.
1400 K Street, N.W.
Washington, DC 20005
www.appi.org

Library of Congress Cataloging-in-Publication Data
Horowitz, Mardi Jon, 1934–
    Treatment of stress response syndromes / Mardi J. Horowitz.
      p. ; cm.
    Includes bibliographical references and index.
    ISBN 1-58562-107-2 (alk. paper)
      1. Stress (Psychology) 2. Stress management. 3. Post-traumatic stress
disorder—Treatment. 4. Life change events.   I. Title.
    [DNLM: 1. Stress, Psychological—therapy. 2. Life Change Events. 3. Stress Disorders,
Post-Traumatic—therapy. WM 172 H816t 2002]
    RC455.4.S87 H67 2002
    155.9'042—dc21
                                                                                2002071115

British Library Cataloguing in Publication Data
A CIP record is available from the British Library.

For Carol, with love

Contents

Preface

This book covers treatment for mental disorders precipitated by the experience of traumatic life events. The basic principles involve understanding symptom formations and the treatment that can lead to resolution of the causes of protracted distress. These principles are grounded in clinical research, a theoretical synthesis of which has been presented in detail elsewhere (Horowitz 1998, 2001). In the present work, the goal is a brief, thorough coverage of an integrated treatment that follows biopsychosocial models and amalgamates different types of therapy.

I have avoided the approach of using chapters as containers of different diagnoses, such as posttraumatic stress, acute stress, adjustment, and other disorders. Instead, I have organized the book by stages of treatment, because essential explanatory principles encompass a range of diagnostic entities; it is easier for clinicians to understand actions based on these principles than to consult and study guidelines for each separate disorder (Marshall et al. 1999). To complement the focus on broad principles, such as those that govern the formation of intrusive and avoidant symptoms, this book emphasizes the importance of explaining a disorder through individualized case formulation. The process for doing this, configurational analysis, is described and illustrated. This integrative approach leads to the development of effective treatment plans and will relate well with what the clinician already knows.

Treating stress response syndromes requires that the clinician listen to stories that are sometimes quite devastating. It is my hope that this book will provide therapists with the necessary tools to support and foster coping skills in their patients as they move through their therapeutic journey: reasons to hope for improvement, courage in facing the repercussions of traumatic events, and the emotional stamina and knowledge needed to find a route to adaptive change.

Acknowledgments

I have been very well supported in scientific studies on the psychological effects of stress by the University of California San Francisco, the National Institute of Mental Health, the John D. and Catherine T. MacArthur Foundation, and the Center for Advanced study in the Behavioral Sciences at Stanford University. Sharing the work and development of ideas were many assistants, associates, patients, and trainees. My principal colleagues were (in alphabetical order) George Bonnano, Gordon Bauer, John Conger, Paul Crits-Christoff, Catherine DeWitt, Tracy Eells, Robert Emde, Matthew Erdelyi, Mary Ewert, Nigel Field, Bram Fridhandler, Jess Ghannam, Dianna Hartley, Are Holen, Michael Hoyt, Nancy Kaltreider, Peter Knapp, Helena Kreamer, Janice Krupnick, Lester Luborsky, Norman Mages, Henry Markman, Charles Marmar, Andreas Mearecker, Erhard Mergenthaler, Tom Merluzzi, Aubrey Metcalf, Constance Milbrath, Dana Redington, Steven Reidbord, Robert Rosenbaum, Peter Salovey, Bryna Siegel, Jerome Singer, Alan Skolnikof, David Spiegel, Charles Stinson, Clyde Sugahara, Eva Sundin, Sandra Tunis, Robert Wallerstein, Daniel Weiss, Nancy Wilner, and Hans Znoj. Lee Jones and Owen Wolkowitz read the manuscript and provided useful additions. Carol Horowitz edited the manuscript and Margarite Salinas compiled it; I am most grateful. At American Psychiatric Publishing, Inc., the able editorial team was Pam Harley, Martin Lynds, Anne Barnes, and Ann Eng.

Theoretically and psychotherapeutically, I am especially indebted to the brief psychodynamic and interpersonal approaches of Basch (1980), Caplan (1961), Klerman and Weissman (1993), Luborsky (1984), Malan (1979), Mann (1973), Parad et al. (1976), Sifneos (1972), and Strupp and Binder (1984); to the cognitive-behavioral and integrative approaches of Beck (1976), Foa and Kozak (1988), Marks et al. (1998), Meichenbaum (1977), and Wachtel (1977); and to the work of others summarized in Follette et al. (1993).

CHAPTER 1

Orientation and Treatment Goals

This book emphasizes the importance of individual case formulation and an integrative approach to psychotherapy (Horowitz 1997a, 1997b, 1998, 1999). The focus is on the treatment of disorders caused by stressor life events involving loss, trauma, and terror. Cardinal symptoms in such stress response syndromes include emotional pangs of distressing intensity coupled with intrusive images and ideas as well as maladaptive avoidances and emotional numbing. These symptoms cross diagnostic categories.

The denial and intrusive states that characterize stress response syndromes are deflections from a person's usual sense of conscious equilibrium. Because avoidance behavior is so common in stress response syndromes, attention to defensive coping and resistances to treatment is important. An integrative approach is valuable: it combines a psychodynamic understanding of control of emotion with useful cognitive-behavioral and pharmacological treatment principles and techniques.

An integrative approach to the treatment of stress response syndromes considers three major areas of mental activity. One is the set of processes that activates emotions, especially affective alarms such as fear. This set of processes is closely linked with somatic physiology and the conditioned associations that occur between perceptual or ideational stimuli and reactive arousals. The second area has to do with activation of trains of conscious thought and preconscious information processing. Dysfunctional

1

beliefs are sometimes used by a person to explain why a distressing event affected him or her. These dysfunctional beliefs lead to repetitive maladaptive behavioral patterns and hence are important to clarify and revise. A third set of mental activities maintains self-organization and a sense of affiliation with others. Maladaptive schemas of relationship interactions may impair social functioning. Identity and relationships may need to change as a result of experiencing stressor life events and the new realities they create.

EMOTIONAL RESPONSES

The important emotional reactions in stress response syndromes consist of 1) a sense of numbness that may be present when denial symptoms are prominent, and 2) its opposite, pangs of strong emotion that accompany other intrusive symptoms, such as a piercing recollection of traumatic images. Numbness is not simply an absence of emotions; it is a felt sense of being remote, muffled, or stifled. The individual may actually feel surrounded by a layer of insulation. Emotional blunting may alter the person's patterns of interaction with important support systems within family life, friendship, and work relations. Members of the person's support network may be offended by these changes in the nature of their relationship and may withdraw, thus reducing social supports just when they are most needed.

Increased escape activity may be used during denial states to numb emotionality. Such escape activity may include excessive engagement in work, sports, or sexual activities. The constant preoccupation with activity jams thinking and feeling channels to such a degree that ideas and emotions related to the stressful event are stifled. Substances such as drugs, alcohol, or nicotine may be used excessively for similar purposes, to quell intrusive states and promote disavowal and emotional numbing.

The opposite experience, pangs of strong emotion, becomes familiar to the person under stress. Such emotion occurs in an intense wave that seems almost unbearable at its peak. The person comes to know that these peaks will be followed by a reduction in intensity that makes it possible to live through this difficult period.

Intrusive emotional states contain reenactments of stressor events and fantasized responses. These compulsive repetitions may take place as a pattern of action and/or occur consciously as memory. A repetition can range from a minor fragment of a larger complex to a complete reliving of the event as if in real time.

One emotional aspect of intrusive states stems from the process of associating alarm emotions with topics other than, but still in some way connected with, the stressor events. Through such overgeneralizations, situations that are usually neutral may be infused with fear, anger, or sadness. In normal reactions to stressor events, a gradual diminution of such reactions occurs through a process termed *desensitization*. In abnormal reactions, however, a persistent or intermittent highly alarmed reaction occurs.

COGNITIVE RESPONSES

During denial phases, disavowal of the meanings of the traumatic event, constriction of the range of thought, and avoidance of trauma-related places, memories, or activities are often prominent. Sometimes a contrived continuation of life as usual contains an altered subjective quality: the person continues thinking about the same topics in the same way as before the stressor event. The person, however, may also feel like an automaton—one who is carrying out habitual patterns that may now be inappropriate. When accompanied by emotional numbing, this automatic repetition of habits leads to a devitalized and joyless manner of living life.

In contrast, during intrusive phases of response, the person can associate other stimuli or topics of thought with stress-related topics, thus priming repetitive memories or ruminations about the stressor event. The stressor theme then becomes both difficult to dispel and difficult to think through to a point of decision, acceptance, and completion. The person may be aware of an overgeneralization of associative links to the stressor event, and that, too, may feel inappropriate to the current and actual situation.

SELF-RELATIONAL RESPONSES

Stressor events present a person with stimuli that drastically conflict with his or her inner schemas. For example, a person expects a limb, an eye, or a body organ to always be present, both functionally and as a part of his or her self-image. If the person loses a body part or undergoes an amputation, a safe world can become a zone of terror. Almost invariably, the conflict between the new reality and the person's inner model of the world has a serious impact on the person's identity and sense of affiliation in relationships. This persists until inner schemas are gradually modified to accord with new and unmodifiable realities. Until that modification is accomplished, the person may experience identity diffusion or chaotic shifts in his or her conscious sense of personal identity, depersonalization, derealization, dissociation, and a sense of being totally abandoned by others.

TREATMENT GOALS

The goal of treatment is to help the person achieve an adaptive emotional equilibrium, process the meanings of the stressor events, and reschematize his or her identity and relationships. The initial aim is to assist the patient so that he or she is neither emotionally blunted nor emotionally flooded. In general, therapists attempt to help people reach a restored sense of safety—a state in which they can use optimum skills in decision making, engage in adaptive coping, and be able to make rational preparations for the future. The focus includes efforts to restore a realistic concept of the self as stable, coherent, competent, and worthwhile, with a sense of competence in work, community, family, and personal functions.

These goals should include plans for protecting the patient from dangers—for example, accidents (from inattention and slowed reaction time), inappropriate decisions (made on the basis of erroneous beliefs or compulsive repetitions), social stigmatization (as a consequence of loss, injury, culpability, or victimization), demoralization or suicide (due to impaired sense of identity and meaning), and disruption of chemophysiology (from prolonged release of stress hormones, fatigue, substance abuse, or excessive use of medications).

This book serves as a general guideline that can be used with several diagnoses when the symptomatic presentation has been precipitated by a recent and personally serious stressor event. Such diagnoses include acute stress disorder, posttraumatic stress disorder, adjustment disorder, major depressive disorder, generalized anxiety disorder, and complicated grief disorder. The following three case examples illustrate, for the beginning clinician, some types of patients that would benefit from the treatment described in this book.

CASE EXAMPLES

Laura

Laura, a 19-year-old woman, lived with her parents and 14-year-old sister while she attended college. On a family automobile trip, their car was struck head on by a drunk driver, killing both her parents. Laura and her sister were hospitalized for bruises and lacerations but were released after 2 days. Laura took care of her younger sister for 2 weeks, then arrangements were made for the sister to live with an aunt and uncle. Laura moved into a group apartment with other college students. During this transition period and for an additional 6 weeks, Laura seemed to be her normal self.

Eight weeks after the crash and funeral for her parents, Laura began to feel extremely tense, sad, and empty. She experienced uncontrolled episodes of sobbing and engaged in tirades of rage directed at the drunk driver. She had intrusive memories of the accident and the funeral. She felt unable to cope with schoolwork and was irritable and remote from her roommates.

Laura's roommates referred her to student health, and from there she was referred to a psychotherapist. She was diagnosed as having an acute stress disorder. The clinician remarked that Laura might have a turbulent period of mourning ahead of her and that she could go into that passage with the therapist's support. Laura sobbed in response to this statement but expressed gratitude for the offer; she tended to have a hopeful attitude toward the treatment.

Gus

Gus, a 25-year-old man, had been stabbed by an unknown and apparently psychotic assailant when he answered his door. Roommates quickly called the paramedics. Gus lost consciousness in the ambulance and awoke in the recovery room after surgery. He had required emergency removal of a torn and hemorrhagic kidney. Three weeks later, he was doing well physically but told his surgeon at a follow-up visit that he felt fragile and fearful. He had a weird sense of pervasive numbness about the assault and the loss of his kidney. Gus was referred for a psychiatric consultation.

Gus appeared quite frightened about the idea of telling the therapist about the assault and the surgery. He could hardly speak in answer to a question concerning how he felt about losing his kidney. The consultant told Gus that he seemed to combine a heightened emotional sensitivity with signs of blocking ideas to avoid emotional states that were too intense. The need to process the event was apparent, and a course of psychotherapy with a gradual exploration of topics related to the trauma was agreed on.

Samantha

Samantha, a 55-year-old woman, appeared for a psychiatric consultation at the insistence of her husband. Her mother, age 90, had died of cancer 1 year before. Samantha had been quite close to her mother; they had talked daily by telephone for decades.

After the death of her mother, Samantha consulted clairvoyants in an attempt to communicate with her mother in the spirit world. The expense of these clairvoyants caused friction with her husband, because they were of limited means and he was nearing his age of mandatory retirement. He was disgusted with Samantha's irrationality and derisively handed her a Ouija board that he had purchased "so she could save money by communicating with her mother without clairvoyants." They had an intense and verbally abusive argument.

Samantha felt agitated, depressed, and desperate after this argument. She felt that she no longer loved her husband; she blamed him and decided she might get a divorce. Samantha's husband was startled when she threatened to leave him. He then told her he loved her but was very concerned about her being so sad and irrational. She agreed to a consultation with their primary care physician.

Samantha told the physician that she missed her mother but felt no grief, just an intense yearning to be in communication with her. Life seemed empty and gray without her mother. Samantha exhibited signs of emotional overcontrol, loss of appetite, and dejection. When the physician asked about her mother's death and the funeral, Samantha's thinking became blocked, and she changed the topic. The physician said she wanted Samantha to have the opportunity to work with a therapist and arranged the referral. His diagnosis was major depressive episode related to the loss.

The psychotherapist concurred with the diagnosis after completing an independent evaluation. Samantha showed a passive-aggressive stance with the psychotherapist, although she came to each appointment on time. In the initial few sessions, she spoke more about her husband than about her mother. The therapist began to persist with the suggestion that they discuss the relationship with her mother. When she did so, Samantha entered into an agitated state and seemed slightly confused. The therapist tactfully noted that it seemed to her that Samantha had some unfinished business and that perhaps their further talking would provide a chance for Samantha to deal with this. Samantha accepted this gambit and began to engage in a discussion of her mother's death and its effects on her and her marriage. The therapy was not as brief as initially expected, as Samantha had to proceed slowly; antidepressant medications were added to the treatment.

CONCLUSIONS

The case examples in this chapter illustrate only some of the wide variety of problems that patients with stress response syndromes present to clinicians. Patients, like Samantha, do not always present the precipitating stressor event as their first topic of expression. They fear that telling about the stressor event, even in a treatment context, will be so emotional they will be retraumatized, as in the case example of Gus.

Any stressor event is complicated in that it leads to a cascade of emotionally problematic topics for personal consideration, as it did in Laura's case. The person who experiences traumatic events, at least implicitly and intuitively, anticipates a long period of turbulent emotions as these topics are gradually considered.

Because the patient is often afraid and confused about what is going on, treatment goals include apt evaluation and as much early support as indicated, as well as a readiness to stay the course with the patient.

CHAPTER 2

Evaluation

In real practice, evaluation extends throughout treatment, with the therapist continually reevaluating the patient's progress and the possibilities for further benefit. However, for didactic purposes, we will consider in sequence six stages of treatment: evaluation, initial support, exploration of meanings, improving coping, working through, and termination. Table 2–1 provides an overview of the key therapist and patient activities in these stages.

Evaluation can be very therapeutic in and of itself. The patient feels hopeful if he or she senses the therapist's expertise, understanding, and compassion. In addition, feedback given by the clinician increases the patient's knowledge of what can happen after serious life events. Such feedback often reduces common fears that intrusive symptoms mean incipient insanity or that the intensity of dreaded states of mind will never abate. The combination of the therapist's empathy and knowledge can quickly establish a therapeutic alliance, and that vital ingredient can take the severe edge off the patient's level of distress.

The components of evaluation include 1) the standard psychiatric history with supplemental topics of particular relevance to stress response syndromes; 2) laboratory and other tests, if and when available and indicated; 3) descriptive diagnoses; and 4) formulation of possible explanations for symptom formation as well as obstacles to active adaptive coping processes. Such a formulation then leads to inferences about whether, how, where, and when changes might occur. The result is a plan for treatment.

TABLE 2–1. Stages of treatment for stress response syndromes

Approximate order	Patient activity	Therapist activity	Therapeutic alliance
1. Evaluation	Patient reports events and personal contexts as well as symptoms.	Therapist obtains history; makes diagnoses and early formulations; provides educative information if needed; and discusses treatment indications and options.	Agreement on initial treatment, with hope fostered by expertise and empathy.
2. Initial support	Patient expands story and focuses on how to cope with current stress.	Therapist acts to stabilize states if indicated and establishes preliminary focus (the traumatic event and its meaning to self).	Roles of therapeutic partnership are defined.
3. Exploration of meanings	Patient expands on meaning to self of trauma and its sequelae.	Therapist realigns focus as formulations are revised. If avoidance is maladaptive, therapist counteracts or interprets defensive and warded-off contents. He or she clarifies how intrusive and warded-off emotions and ideas are linked to stressor events and patient's appraisals of them.	Therapeutic alliance deepened by experience of safety. Patient may test therapist to see whether fears of what may happen (e.g., fear of emotional overload) are justified.

TABLE 2–1. Stages of treatment for stress response syndromes *(continued)*

Approximate order	Patient activity	Therapist activity	Therapeutic alliance
4. Improving coping	Patient works on themes previously avoided.	Therapist acts to encourage desensitization of triggers to emotional reactions and helps patient to modify dysfunctional beliefs.	Deeper expression of usually private thoughts and emotions.
5. Working through	Patient revises beliefs and mental structure (reschematizes cognitive maps of identity and relationships).	Therapist helps patient to modify structure of beliefs (reschematization).	Projections and transference reactions are confronted and clarified in relation to the actualities.
6. Termination	Patient considers gains and unfinished issues, as well as how to cope with loss of the therapy.	Therapist clarifies gains and any unfinished issues for the future; and interprets and differentiates any links between termination experiences and stressor-event experiences.	Emphasis is on safe separation.

PSYCHIATRIC HISTORY

Taking a patient's psychiatric history, assessing his or her mental status, and making a diagnosis will be familiar to most clinicians. In evaluating stress response syndromes, one does not deviate from the usual procedures. It should be noted, however, that some patients will find it difficult to discuss the stressor event. In intrusive phases of response, the pangs of emotion and the undermodulated states of mind precipitated by recall of the event may interrupt the flow of information. In denial phases of response, the person may express anxious and depressive signs and symptoms of psychiatric disorders without adequate information about the inciting stressors. In all phases, some distortions of memory may occur (Andrews et al. 1999; Elliott 1997; Kardiner and Spiegel 1947; Spiegel 1997; Williams and Banyard 1999; Wilson and Raphael 1993).

For these reasons, an initial open topics approach is often useful. Such an approach allows the patient to speak at his or her own discretion, thus providing an opportunity for the clinician to observe signs of excessive or underregulated control of emotionality when certain topics emerge. The clinician can use such observations to assess which topics are unresolved as well as to consider the patient's degree of irrationality, distortion, and suppression of recall or response.

The clinician gradually introduces a more structured approach. The questions he or she asks will be specific to the patient's individual situation as well as covering the general topics listed in Table 2–2. Again, these topics represent a stress supplement to the usual topics discussed when taking a psychiatric history.

Usually the telling of one stressor event precipitates a cascade of other information. In taking a history, it is important that the clinician place the trauma within a biological, psychological, and social framework (Kleber et al. 1995; Lindeman 1944). Similar events from the past, personality traits, social supports, and physical factors (e.g., a possible concussion from an auto accident) will all be relevant. The context in which a stressor event occurs is very important.

A history of any previous exposure to traumatic events is important because of two factors: 1) such a history is associated with a higher incidence of posttraumatic stress disorder (PTSD), multiple previous events having the strongest effect (Breslau et al. 1999a); and 2) the person is likely to have special sensitivities, beliefs, and schemas of self as related to others derived from previous exposures, especially if they occurred during formative years.

Personality traits are also important to assess. The configurational analysis method of case formulation, soon to be discussed, is especially

TABLE 2–2.	Important topics in the evaluation of stress response syndromes

1. History of precipitating events
2. Current symptoms and problems, especially those with onset after the stressor event
3. States of mind in which symptoms do and do not occur, and new states or shifts in states experienced since the stressor event
4. Meaning of stressor events to the goals and prior expectations of the patient
5. Past traumatic events and reactions to them
6. Comorbid conditions
7. Usual and present coping strategies
8. Social supports and pressures, especially those changed by the stressor event
9. Substance and medication history, including increased uses after the stressor event
10. Expectations about treatment and how it might work or fail (including the expectation that therapy could be a kind of retraumatization)

helpful in this regard. Negativism, neuroticism, and low self-confidence have all been implicated as possible risk factors for PTSD in epidemiological studies (e.g., Bramsen et al. 2000; Card 1987; McFarlane 1988).

The support systems of the person are vital to assess. Low socioeconomic status increases the likelihood of depressive and other symptoms (Adler et al. 1998). Displacement of anger responses to inappropriate targets of rage, inadequate family cohesion, and an absence of confidants all are likely to reduce the rate of recovery (Hammen et al. 1992).

TESTS

Tests are not yet a routine part of clinical evaluation of the stress response syndromes, but substantial progress is being made in understanding the causation of these disorders. Additions to psychiatric history taking, such as laboratory tests, are likely to become available in the future as a consequence of research advances. I envision that these may include 1) blood tests for levels of adrenal hormones, metabolites of neurotransmitters, and immunological factors that may be altered by stress; 2) brain imaging for abnormalities in specific metabolic sites; and 3) tests of autonomic nervous system responses. In addition to these predictions regarding future physical tests, there are already 4) a variety of self-report and observer rating scales that can be used both in the initial assessment and in tracking levels of subjective or objective distress.

One widely used scale for self-report of intrusive and avoidant symptoms is the Impact of Event Scale (Horowitz et al. 1979; Sundin and Horowitz 2001; Table 2–3). The clinician anchors the scale to experiences related to a particular stressor event or series of events. The scale yields total scores and can be periodically readministered. The author holds the copyright for and gives the reader permission to copy and use this scale. Mean scores from various trauma populations are shown in Table 2–4 (Horowitz et al. 1993).

There are other self- and observer rating scales for specific stressors, for stress response in general, and for highly relevant general symptoms such as anxiety, depression, and somatization. The most recent versions of these instruments can be found in publications (and sometimes the Internet sites) of organizations such as the American Psychiatric Association (www.psych.org), the American Psychological Association (www.apa.org), and the International Society for Traumatic Stress Studies (www.istss.org). Some such scales can be used as a screening method after a large-scale disaster. For example, Breslau et al. (1999b) constructed a 7-question, telephone-administered screening scale for use in identifying possible cases of PTSD.

DIAGNOSIS

Several descriptive diagnoses (DSM-IV; American Psychiatric Association 1994) pertain to stress response syndromes: PTSD, acute stress disorder, adjustment disorder, substance abuse disorder, major depressive episode or disorder, complicated grief disorder, generalized anxiety disorder, panic disorder, and phobic disorder precipitated by stressor events. All may involve symptoms of intrusion and avoidance of stress-related memories and emotions, symptoms already partly illustrated in Table 2–3. Flare-ups of personality problems also may be precipitated by stressor events. Persons with histrionic, narcissistic, and borderline personality disorders often have traumatic events in childhood and are vulnerable to symptoms if and when contextually similar traumas occur.

The frequency of PTSD is illustrated by the following study. In a random epidemiological sample of 1,000 people in a Midwestern United States city, the current rates of full PTSD (all DSM-IV criteria) were assessed. The disorder was found to be present in 2.7% of women and 1.2% of men (Stein et al. 1997). These numbers would have been even larger if all stress response syndromes had been included. Of interest, in this study, is that 60% of the participants had sought help.

The key signs of a stress-induced syndrome are intrusive and avoidant symptoms. Patients with a primary diagnosis of PTSD were compared with

TABLE 2–3. Impact of Event Scale

Name of Subject: _____ Date: _____

Directions: Below is a list of comments made by people about stressful life events and the context surrounding them. Read each item and decide how frequently each item was true for you DURING THE PAST 7 DAYS regarding (insert relevant event) _____. If the item did not occur during the past 7 days, choose the NOT AT ALL option. Circle the number of the response which best describes that item. Please put a circle somewhere after each of the 15 items.

(0) Not at all   (1) Rarely   (3) Sometimes   (5) Often

	Not at all	Rarely	Sometimes	Often
1. I thought about it when I didn't mean to.	0	1	3	5
2. I avoided letting myself get upset when I thought about it or was reminded of it.	0	1	3	5
3. I tried to remove it from memory.	0	1	3	5
4. I had trouble falling asleep or staying asleep because of pictures or thoughts that came into my mind.	0	1	3	5
5. I had waves of strong feelings about it.	0	1	3	5
6. I had dreams about it.	0	1	3	5
7. I stayed away from reminders of it.	0	1	3	5
8. I felt as if it had not happened or was not real.	0	1	3	5
9. I tried not to talk about it.	0	1	3	5
10. Pictures about it popped into my mind.	0	1	3	5
11. Other things kept making me think about it.	0	1	3	5
12. I was aware that I still had a lot of feelings about it, but I didn't deal with them.	0	1	3	5
13. I tried not to think about it.	0	1	3	5
14. Any reminder brought back feelings about it.	0	1	3	5
15. My feelings about it were kind of numb.	0	1	3	5

Source. Reprinted from Horowitz MJ, Wilner N, Alvarez W: "The Impact of Event Scale: A Measure of Subjective Stress." *Psychosomatic Medicine* 41:209–218, 1979. Used with permission.

TABLE 2–4. Impact of Event subscale scores for various trauma populations

Population (author)	Event	N	Weeks, mean (SD)	Intrusion, mean (SD)	Avoidance, mean (SD)
Israeli soldiers with PTSD (Solomon 1989)	1982 Lebanon War	382	52 (—)	17.4 (9.7)	17.7 (12.8)
		285	104 (—)	14.6 (9.5)	16.1 (12.6)
		213	156 (—)	13.0 (9.3)	14.4 (12.3)
Israeli soldiers without PTSD (Solomon 1989)	1982 Lebanon War	334	52 (—)	6.8 (6.2)	8.4 (9.7)
		198	104	4.9	7.0
		116	156 (—)	4.3 (6.0)	6.8 (9.3)
American soldiers with PTSD before phenelzine (Frank et al. 1988)	Vietnam War	11	>500	22.0	19.0
American soldiers with PTSD after phenelzine (Frank et al. 1988)	Vietnam War	12	>500 (—)	9.0 (9.3)	11.0 (6.0)
Disaster victims (Laube 1986)	Earthquake in Kalamata, Greece	83	5 (0)	27.3 (7.5)	21.1 (7.7)
Disaster victims (Foreman 1988)	Plane crash into Sun Valley Mall	17	27 (—)	25.7 (9.8)	21.9 (10.5)
		11	82 (—)	19.4 (10.2)	18.9 (11.4)
Rescue workers (Foreman 1988)	Plane crash into Sun Valley Mall	20	27 (—)	11.8 (10.1)	9.2 (10.4)
		15	82 (—)	8.3 (10.7)	5.2 (7.3)
Female disaster survivors (Steinglass and Gerrity 1990)	Tornado	18	17 (—)	17.9 (7.4)	15.6 (8.9)
		20	68 (—)	8.9 (6.6)	12.0 (10.0)

TABLE 2–4. Impact of Event subscale scores for various trauma populations *(continued)*

Population (author)	Event	N	Weeks, mean (SD)	Intrusion, mean (SD)	Avoidance, mean (SD)
Male disaster survivors (Steinglass and Gerrity 1990)	Tornado	15 / 19	17 (—) / 68 (—)	9.6 (9.0) / 7.0 (8.5)	11.4 (11.5) / 5.4 (7.4)
Family survivors of violence (Amick-McMullan et al. 1989)	Homicide of family member	16	130 (130)	24.6 (—)	16.9 (—)
Rape survivors (Kilpatrick and Veronen 1984)	Rape	23	104 (—)	11.2 (—)	16.0 (—)
Patients with stress response syndromes at treatment onset (Horowitz et al. 1984b)	Death of a parent	35 / 35	26 (20) / 66 (17)	20.1 (7.8) / 8.4 (6.2)	20.8 (10.6) / 6.2 (8.2)
Bereaved nonpatient control subjects (Horowitz et al. 1984b)	Death of a parent	37 / 37	8 (2) / 58 (9)	13.5 (9.5) / 6.9 (7.9)	9.3 (9.6) / 5.8 (8.2)
Surgical tumor patients (Horowitz et al. 1979)	Breast biopsy for possible cancer	68	1 (0)	7.2 (7.5)	7.5 (9.0)
Medical tumor patients (Horowitz et al. 1979)	Cancer diagnosis	54	5 (3)	8.4 (8.2)	9.2 (8.1)
Medical students (Horowitz et al. 1979)	First exposure to and dissection of cadaver	69	2 (0)	4.0 (4.4)	6.0 (6.3)

a matched sample of patients with a primary diagnosis of major depressive disorder (Reynolds and Brewin 1999). Assessment with the Impact of Event Scale, which measures intrusive and avoidant symptoms by self-report on a 15-item set of ratings, resulted in the finding that levels of frequency of such symptoms were similar in both diagnostic groups. Intrusive and avoidant symptoms are also found in acute stress disorder, complicated grief disorder, and many adjustment disorders.

Denial and Intrusive Symptoms

Denial symptoms include emotional numbness and excessive cognitive inhibitions. Intrusive symptoms include hypervigilance, sleep and dream disturbances, pangs of unwanted feeling, unbidden images, and intrusive–repetitive thoughts. These symptoms may coalesce into a state of mind. Denial and intrusive states may occur in phases, as illustrated in Figure 2–1. These common symptoms are summarized in Table 2–5.

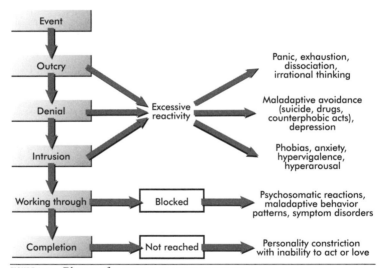

FIGURE 2–1.　Phases of response to stressor events.

It is not uncommon for a person to be in a shimmering state in which he or she experiences both denial and intrusion. Patients often experience this state during the phase of working through the conflicted meanings and implications of a stressor event. The patient might experience intrusions of some themes but ward off others (or aspects of a theme that occur as an intrusion).

TABLE 2-5. Symptoms and signs commonly seen in all stress response syndromes during denial and intrusive states

	Denial states	Intrusive states
Perception and attention	Daze Selective inattention Inability to appreciate significance of stimuli	Hypervigilance, startle reactions Sleep and dream disturbances
Consciousness of ideas and feelings related to the event	Amnesia (complete or partial) Noncontemplation of topics that ought to be considered because of implications of the stressor event	Intrusive–repetitive thoughts, emotions, and behaviors (illusions, pseudohallucinations, nightmares, unbidden images, ruminations) Feeling pressured, confused, or disorganized when thinking about event-related themes
Information processing	Disavowal of meanings of current stimuli in some way associated with the event Loss of realistic sense of appropriate connection with the ongoing world Constriction of range of thought Inflexibility of purpose Major use of fantasies to counteract real conditions	Overgeneralization of stimuli so that they seem related to the event Preoccupation with event-related themes with inability to concentrate on other topics
Emotional attributes	Numbness	Emotional attacks or pangs of affect related to the event or to reminders
Action patterns	Frantic overactivity Withdrawal Failure to decide how to respond to consequences of event	Compulsive repetitions of actions associated with the event or of search for lost persons or situations

TABLE 2–5. Symptoms and signs commonly seen in all stress response syndromes during denial and intrusive states *(continued)*

	Denial states	Intrusive states
Somatic attributes	Excessive sleeping; lethargy; hibernative states	Altered activities, usually hyperarousal of the autonomic nervous system with felt sensations such as bowel pain, diarrhea, or constipation; fatigue; headache; muscle pain, cramps, or tremors; intense startle reactions; palpitations, high pulse rate, or hypertension; restlessness

The model of outcry, denial, intrusion, and working-through phases is useful in understanding the variety of changing individual responses to stress. However, it should not be concretized into a rigid expectation of everyone. Many possible patterns of response exist, and each person's pattern will necessarily differ—both phasically and temporally—from that of other individuals.

Given such individual variation, both clinicians and patients will have questions about what constitutes a disorder and what represents a normal turbulence that will subside without treatment. Usually this question can be answered in several ways. First, patients themselves often will have an intuitive sense of whether they are experiencing a resolving or nonresolving response. Second, the passage of time is a vital index of normal response and disorder: the person who demonstrates extreme acute symptoms over a long period of time is more likely to have PTSD (Yehuda and McFarlane 1995).

Comorbidities

Comorbidities are very common in stress response syndromes (Kessler et al. 1995). Several important mechanisms are involved. Prior traumas may have led to a personality disorder. Personality problems may make the person more prone to a stress-induced disorder, especially when current circumstances are linked with memories or unconscious schematizations from earlier life traumas. Substance abuse also makes a person more likely to experience stressor events and less able to cope. In addition, people are more likely to relapse into more substance abuse under stress-induced distress (Brady et al. 2001; Jacobsen et al. 2001).

Biopsychosocial Frameworks

Because of variability in individual responses and the high frequency of comorbidity, this author's primarily psychological model of stress response syndromes (Horowitz 1976), as condensed into Figure 2–1, has been challenged. Some feel that this model leads to social stigmatization because it overemphasizes psychopathological reactions (Shephard 2001). Others call into question the idea that PTSD represents a maladaptive intensification or distortion of normal tendencies such as conditioned fear responsivity, active memory storage of important and incompletely processed memories, intrusive repetition of such memories, and excessive control of information processing to avoid recapitulation of traumatic feelings. Instead, these authors emphasize the role of abnormal mechanisms such as biological deficiencies that may have preexisted or been induced by traumas (Yehuda and McFarlane 1995). Both the social and the biological challenges are useful; we should employ a biopsychosocial framework in developing our understanding of diagnoses. Our diagnostic system has changed over time and will continue to change as we gain explanatory theory.

Multiaxial Diagnosis

As already mentioned, syndromes such as acute stress disorder, PTSD, and adjustment disorder are classified as Axis I (clinical) disorders in DSM-IV. Complicated grief belongs in such a grouping (Horowitz et al. 1997; Jacobs 1999; Prigerson et al. 1995). These are the syndromes most clearly caused by stressors. Other Axis I disorders may not have been present prior to an inciting serious stress event—or, if present, they may have worsened to such a degree that treatment for a stress response syndrome is indicated, at least as an adjunct to other treatment components. Such disorders include substance abuse, phobic anxiety, generalized anxiety, panic, and major depressive disorders, as well as (more rarely, in my experience) reactive psychoses. Furthermore, a psychiatric hospitalization for any disorder can for some patients be a traumatic experience, leading to posttraumatic symptoms and requiring treatment to reduce the traumatic memories. Because of this complexity, and because of comorbidities, the use of multiple and multiaxial diagnoses is valuable in the treatment of stress response syndromes.

It is useful to first assign several Axis I (clinical symptom disorder) diagnoses and then to assign a personality disorder diagnosis (Axis II) if indicated. It is also possible to indicate a personality style without assigning a personality disorder diagnosis; some styles (e.g., histrionic, narcissistic) may predict expectable difficulties in establishing a therapeutic alliance. Injuries sustained during a traumatic event are highly relevant and are diagnosed in Axis III (general medical conditions). Seemingly mild concussions are relevant as well, because they often have chronic effects (Trimble 1981). Psychosocial and environmental problems (Axis IV) are pertinent and central in many responses to wartime and natural disasters (Maskin 1941). The global assessment of functioning (Axis V) should be considered as well.

Although roughly half of patients with stress response symptoms may have personality problems tangled in a web of symptom formation and coping strategies, these patients do not usually fit well into a single personality disorder diagnostic category in Axis II of DSM-IV. Complex issues of character and genetically determined temperament play a role in stress response syndromes (Kendler et al. 1999). For this reason, the key prerequisite to treatment planning is formulation—formulation addresses the reasons for symptom formation and the causes of insufficient coping. Diagnosis is essential, but it is not enough. Formulation provides the individualization that is required for optimal treatment.

FORMULATION AND TREATMENT PLANNING

As just mentioned, individualized case formulation is the best route from assessment and diagnosis to optimum treatment planning. Individuals have combinations of strengths as well as weaknesses; they have life goals and plans affected by the stressor events, as well as varied concepts of identity and affiliations. They exhibit different symptoms, moods, and defenses in different states of mind. Assessing these factors means considering configurations of states, beliefs, and roles of relating to the world. The approach I propose for learning what topics should be addressed by the therapist, what states to look for when working on such topics, and how to help the patient stabilize his or her sense of identity and relatedness is called *configurational analysis* (Horowitz 1997).

Configurational Analysis Method of Case Formulation

Configurational analysis is a systematic method of case formulation that consists of five steps (summarized in Tables 2–6 and 2–7). Each step is based on clinical research about what clinicians can reliably agree upon (Horowitz 1987, 1997, 1998). After each step is considered, the inferences are integrated and treatment planned according to the individualized view of what has happened, what has caused it, and what can change to improve the future for the patient.

In this approach, the clinician first looks at the *phenomena* and selects the key symptoms and problems to be explained. He or she then describes *states* in which both intrusive and avoidant phenomena occur. These may include *dreaded* states of intrusive images and horror and less distressing and more *defensive* states of denial and numbing. These dreaded and defensive states can be contrasted with *desired* states of restored equilibrium. Sometimes defensive states represent protective compromises; at other times they may represent maladaptive, symptomatic, and/or problematic compromises. The compromise is between what the person wants—to experience and master emotional responses—and what the person fears—being overwhelmed by intense and unending distress.

In the third step, the clinician notes the *key unresolved topics and defenses*. The fourth step adds *self–other beliefs that lead to identity and relationships*. Pathogenic stress-induced shifts into such roles as degraded, incompetent, abandoned, shamed, scorned, abused, and unworthy are identified. Often it is helpful to take a key unresolved topic and fit pertinent roles into a configuration of relationship schemas. For example, such a topic may be the loss of a spouse. A configuration of schemas in this case would include the desired roles of regaining a good affiliation, the dreaded roles brought on

TABLE 2–6.	Steps of formulation for stress response syndromes: configurational analysis method

1. **Phenomena**
   Select the symptoms and problems that need to be explained and describe the stressor events that precipitated them.

2. **States of mind**
   Describe states in which the symptoms and problems do and do not occur. Indicate triggers to intrusive and other problematic or dreaded states. Include states of avoidance and impairments to achieving positive states of mind. Describe any maladaptive cycles of states.

3. **Topics of concern and defensive control processes**
   Describe unresolved stress-related topics and how they evolve to problematic states. Identify persisting dysfunctional beliefs. Infer how enduring beliefs mismatch with the newly perceived reality because of the effects of the stressor events. Describe how expression and contemplation of these unresolved topics is obscured. Infer how avoidant operations are used to ward off dreaded states.

4. **Identity and relationships**
   For each recurrent state, infer roles of self and others and their schematized transactions. Describe desired and dreaded role relationship models. Infer how compromise role relationship models ward off danger. Describe repetitive dysfunctional beliefs about roles and cause-and-effect sequences.

5. **Integration and treatment planning**
   Consider problematic biopsychosocial interactions and how to ameliorate them. Explain how schemas of self and other lead to problematic states and how pathogenic defenses prevent resolution of topics of concern. Examine factors that operate to prolong symptoms and suggest how they might be counteracted. From this formulation, predict how to facilitate change. Plan how to stabilize working states and prevent pathologically impulsive actions. Consider how and when to modify beliefs and behaviors, alter social supports, and design treatments for biological impairments.

Source. Adapted from Horowitz 1997.

by the worst imagined consequences of being bereft, and the compromise roles, which are neither as good as desired nor as bad as dreaded. The configuration might contain both a problematic compromise—for example, the self as helpless and needing to anxiously cling to any available dominant figure—and a protective compromise—such as the self as a loner who will never again need a relationship that might be lost.

In the fifth step, the inferences and explanations are used to develop an *integration and treatment plan*. This integration includes a linkage between states, unresolved topics, and core role relationship models. The clinician attempts to explain how dysfunctional beliefs, as incorporated into schemas

TABLE 2–7.	Worksheet for configurational analysis

1. **Phenomena**
   Main symptoms and problems:
   Stressor events that precipitated the above:
2. **States of mind**
   Desired:
   Dreaded:
   Problematic compromise:
   Protective compromise:
   Triggers to dreaded states:
   Maladaptive state cycle:
3. **Topics of concern and defenses**
   Unresolved stress related topics:
   Persisting dysfunctional beliefs:
   Enduring beliefs that mismatch with stressor news:
   Ways that expressions of unresolved topics are obscured:
   Ways in which avoidances can ward off dreaded states:
4. **Identity and relationships**
   Roles of self, other, and schematized transactions:
       Desired:
       Dreaded:
       Problematic compromise:
       Protective compromise:
5. **Integration and treatment planning**
   Biological factors:
   Social, cultural factors:
   What can change and how:
   Program components and plan:

of self and other, lead to problematic and dreaded states. Such an integration also includes inferences about how defenses may shift schemas of self and other to alter emotionality, as well as how excessive inhibition of information processing might be preventing the resolution of key topics of concern. In planning treatment, the clinician considers how to enhance coping capacity and support to heighten a sense of safety so that extreme avoidances can be set aside.

An important aspect of formulation is the therapist's evaluation of the patient's mental structure of beliefs that organize identity and affiliation in relationships. Patients who are more vulnerable to losing identity coherence, who use reality-distorting defenses, and who have explosive shifts in their relationships usually require slower, more supportive exploration of their problems. Some of the signs that may indicate the need for slower and more supportive work with a patient are listed in Table 2–8.

TABLE 2–8.	Signs that reveal a patient's limited capacity for rapid psychotherapeutic work

1. Shows frequent and surprising shifts in state of mind
2. Displays contradictory views of a specific other person from one moment to the next
3. Displays extreme emotional reactions (e.g., rage) to minor hassles in the therapy arrangements
4. Yields easily to impulses
5. Uses highly distorted information processing to regulate self-esteem
6. Does not read the therapist's communications well, which can give the therapist a sense of uneasiness
7. Reacts to therapist's statements as if they are very insulting and jarring

CASE EXAMPLES

Often, clinicians are more comfortable with diagnosis than with case formulation. For brevity, the following case examples focus on formulation issues. The first example illustrates how a stressor event can become entangled with preexisting personality issues.

Harold

While traveling on business in another country, Harold and his wife escaped a hotel fire with minor smoke inhalation injuries. Their schedule was disrupted. Harold and his wife agreed that she would return home at once while Harold rescheduled his local appointments.

In the ensuing days, as he engaged in his business activities, Harold felt unreal and numb. He also experienced a state in which he became too talkative and attention seeking with the women he encountered in business. Five nights after the fire, Harold awakened from a nightmare, screaming, "Mommy, Mommy." During the sixth day, he was tense, felt anxious, and had a sense of chaos about his life roles. He canceled his business appointments, flew home, and sought professional help.

On evaluation, Harold was found to have intrusive memories of the fire, of seeing his wife off at the airport, and of being embarrassed by his engagement with business women. He felt phobic and avoided planning future business travel even though his work depended on it. He experienced nearly constant tension and had a few episodes of hyperventilation.

Harold received a diagnosis of acute stress disorder. He was inferred to have undermodulated states organized by vulnerable self-concepts and roles of dependency in relationships. Although these person schemas had been present (but latent) before the trauma, they were reactivated by the stressor context. It was decided to focus a brief therapy on the topic of the fire and his subsequent reactions. Part of this focus would be how and why the fire and its sequelae led to an activation of Harold's schema of feeling like a needy boy who required maternal attention and felt abandoned and frightened without it.

The task of restoring equilibrium was rapidly accomplished. After 2 weeks, Harold's intrusive, avoidant, and hyperarousal symptoms had diminished, although he still felt vulnerable and lacking in his usual verve and self-confidence. Additional therapy sessions then focused on aspects of dependency and counterphobic negations of dependency in his relationship with his wife. This work increased Harold's sense of self-confidence and identity coherence. It enabled him to engage more mutually with his wife than he had been able to do before the event. He recovered all of his pretraumatic functional levels and felt even better about his capacity for intimate affiliation.

Harold's trauma was minor in comparison with that in the next case example, in which a cascade of traumatic realizations were experienced in the wake of an unfortunate accident. The following case example illustrates denial of important topics brought up by a stressor event. It also illustrates the longer time period that was needed to assimilate a more extreme stressor event than the one experienced by Harold.

Sophia

Sophia made an excellent living as a sought-after model until a sudden car accident resulted in severe injuries that caused permanent blindness and required amputation of one of her legs. She also emerged with severe facial scarring. Sophia spent weeks in the hospital and then months in a convalescent home.

Initially, she did not allow herself to be aware of her blindness; she would not discuss the topic. She did, however, think and talk about the loss of her leg. Her lack of recognition of her blindness was astonishing to staff members, given that she required constant assistance in many functions.

As described in more detail elsewhere (Horowitz 1998), Sophia's sense of identity had not shifted to accommodate the terrible news of her altered body. She repeatedly asked staff members when she could schedule her modeling appointments. Only after weeks had passed did she communicate about being blind; the topic of her facial disfigurement and loss of a career required an even longer period to be broached. Three months after the accident, she finally agreed to have a psychiatric consultation. She was diagnosed as having PTSD and accepted a recommendation for psychotherapy.

Formulation focused on the changes in her body and their social implications. An extreme discord was present between Sophia's internal mental model of herself and her physical alterations. Mourning and identity growth would take a long time. A long-term supportive and expressive psychotherapy was planned. In the context of this therapy, Sophia required 2 years to recover psychological equilibrium and to develop an identity that was coherent with her altered bodily functioning and social opportunities. She learned new self-concepts through a variety of means, including identification with the effective roles and positive attitudes she observed in various health professionals. She trained as a rehabilitation therapist specializing in music therapy. Later she married, and still later became a teacher who trained music therapists.

The following examples of Harry and Frank illustrate how the steps of formulation can be used to organize the information derived from evaluation interviews.

Harry

Harry, a truck driver, picked up a female hitchhiker while carrying a load of pipe to another destination. His truck ran off the road and some of the pipe lurched forward, piercing the unarmored section of the cab where the passenger was riding. The woman was killed instantly. Harry received a diagnosis of PTSD.

Phenomena to Explain

Four weeks after the accident, Harry had a nightmare in which mangled bodies appeared, and he awoke with an anxiety attack. Throughout the following days, he had recurrent, intense, intrusive images of the dead woman's body. These images, together with ruminations about the woman, were accompanied by anxiety attacks of growing severity. Harry also developed a phobia about driving, and his habitual weekend drinking increased to nightly use of alcohol. He had temper outbursts in response to minor frustrations and found it difficult to concentrate at work.

States of Mind

Harry experienced a dreaded state of horror, a problematic state of rage, and a defensive numbing state when he contemplated the traumatic event and its consequences. The state of horror occurred intrusively, with pangs of guilt and shame, and was difficult to dispel. It was triggered by any stimulus that could possibly be associated with the woman's death. The state of rage was also intrusive, even explosive, and therefore problematic. It was triggered by any work-related accusations or domestic demands made on him. An avoidant–numb state was preferable for defensive reasons. Harry's maladaptive cycle ranged from a state of horror in response to reminders of the accident to rage in which he blamed any currently irritating person, to avoidance. He fostered avoidant–numb states through his excessive use of alcohol.

Topics of Concern and Defensive Control Processes

Harry's sense of self-control was markedly reduced by the states of horror and rage, and he worried about what this meant for his mental stability. Other topics of concern were the implications of the accident and the death of his passenger. To avoid these topics, Harry did not think about the event or his work. He used alcohol to blot out ideas and feelings about the accident and to stifle thoughts about its future implications to his life. This avoidance increased Harry's risk of having another traumatic event because it altered his attention, reaction times, and ability to adapt.

Identity and Relationships

Harry desired to feel safe, competent, moral, and respected by others. Instead, he experienced dreaded states involving contrary beliefs about himself as an aggressor and transgressor who caused the accident. As a defensive compromise, he viewed himself as a victim, one who was unfairly blamed. This defense did not quite work. Harry's self-esteem was degraded by feeling stigmatized for breaking the rules, picking up a female hitch-hiker, and driving carelessly.

Harry also felt guilty about being glad that he had survived, as if this relief were an aggressive act and that by magical thinking he had chosen his passenger to be the one who had to die. The magical thinking functioned as a dysfunctional belief about roles in the sequence of cause and effect.

Integration and Treatment Planning

In addition to the above-stated psychological factors, Harry probably had a biological inclination to become addicted to alcohol; a combination of anxiety, depressive, and drinking disorders occurred with unusual frequency in his family. His surrounding culture also tended to support alcohol as a way of coping with stress-induced distress. To help him change, group support for abstinence would be suggested.

In planning treatment, it would be important to note that at treatment onset, Harry could not tolerate the shame, guilt, and horror aroused by consideration of his memories and their implications. He felt too out of control and desperate to contemplate these themes. To maintain some sense of equilibrium and to prevent entry into these dreaded states of mind, he inhibited thought and blunted his feelings with alcohol. Although the alcohol abuse led to problems, it was also Harry's way of avoiding dreaded states. With increased social support, a therapeutic alliance, and encouragement to think about the unresolved emotional topics, Harry could be expected to gain a sense of mastery and self-confidence in experiencing unpleasant emotional states.

The first goal of treatment was to stabilize Harry's state of mind and reduce his alcohol abuse. This involved improvement in sleep and reduction of fatigue and anxiety. An expert helping relationship and a focus on dose-by-dose coping would support these aims. It was expected that the therapeutic situation would rapidly counteract Harry's demoralization and state instability. If this did not occur, use of a selective serotonin reuptake inhibitor would be considered. Finally, in addition to individual psychotherapy, a Twelve-Step group–oriented program to stop alcohol abuse would be part of the recommended treatment.

After initial state stabilization, psychotherapy would focus on improvement in expressive communication. For each topic of concern, Harry's core functional and dysfunctional beliefs were to be explored and any dysfunctional beliefs countered with realistic alternatives. Once self-confidence and control were restored, a time of termination would be set. These plans would be upgraded as additional information was gained in treatment and the individualized formulation was revised.

As in the case of Harry, the case example of Frank illustrates how formulation leads to treatment planning.

Frank

Frank was a 25-year-old lifeguard at a neighborhood pool. On one busy summer day, the pool was full of children and adolescents. In addition to the many people in the water, unruly episodes were occurring on the deck. Frank was quite busy and realized that he was so overloaded with demands for his attention that he could not be sure that everyone was safe. Frank blew his whistle and ordered the pool cleared.

To his horror, there was an inert body at the bottom of the pool. He dived in at once and brought a small, limp, nonbreathing form to the deck. Frank began cardiopulmonary resuscitation. This failed to revive the small boy, who was later pronounced dead. Overcome with remorse, Frank went to the funeral of the deceased child. He was greeted with many angry scowls and became upset by the grief-stricken faces of the child's parents. On evaluation, 6 months later, Frank was diagnosed as having PTSD.

Phenomena to Explain

Frank went through turbulent periods of remorse, insomnia, attacks of anxiety, guilt, and shame, and he developed a dread of dying. He quit his job, had difficulty concentrating, and avoided pools, children, and the neighborhood where he had worked as a lifeguard.

Six months after the event, Frank began having frightening nightmares with visual images of a dead body in a pool, a blurred face of a child, and angry faces of adults. He was preoccupied with feelings of remorse that disturbed his concentration at his new job. He had outbursts of anger with companions. These intrusions occurred despite his efforts to avoid them.

States of Mind

Frank could not sustain interest in his career or recreational activities. A desired state of productive working or focused concentration could seldom be stabilized. Instead, he felt that everything in his world was cloaked in fog. At times he had a dreaded undermodulated state that bordered on panic— he felt like he was about to die. At other times he was preoccupied with angry memories of the pool owners or was irritable in general. These states were markedly different from his usual amiability and enthusiasm before the drowning.

Topics of Concern and Defensive Control Processes

Frank was remote and apathetic when pressed for details about his current feelings. It was difficult to clarify the subjects that seemed to cause his most dreaded states. This difficulty was ameliorated as the therapist communicated empathic and compassionate recognition of Frank's suffering. Frank was then able to move toward exploration of an important topic: he had entangled realistic and fantasized aspects of his responsibilities as a lifeguard.

He felt horribly guilty; it was necessary for the therapist to get beyond Frank's surface statements that he had already worked through this issue. He used warding-off rationalizations by saying, "It was the fault of others."

Identity and Relationships

Frank viewed himself with antithetical sets of self-concepts. His dreaded sense of identity was as an irresponsible, negligent, self-centered caretaker. His desired sense of identify was as a truly caring person who was competent at protecting others. In problematic compromise states, Frank reduced his guilty feelings by externalizing blame onto the pool directors, who did not care enough to hire additional lifeguards or control the number of people allowed to use the pool. In his protective compromise states, he saw himself as a loner with only foggy connections to others.

Integration and Treatment Planning

No significant biological and social factors complicated his case; Frank was not surrounded by social stigmatization, although in his own thoughts he felt enormously responsible for the child's death. Psychotherapy was seen as the treatment of choice. It was expected that the stages of initial support and improving coping would go quickly. During those stages, the plan was to focus on the current stressor.

Frank was at an intrusive phase of response, with many continuing avoidant responses. During the initial support stage, the treatment plan focused on communicating empathetic acceptance of him as suffering and worthy of help. Exploration of meanings and working through were expected to be the most central and longest stages of treatment. During those stages, one topic that emerged as unresolved and important was Frank's rage at the pool managers for putting him in an overly demanding situation. This was linked to the theme of his own guilt. Relegation of blame was the umbrella connecting topic.

As it happened, exploring the anger and guilt topic led to a negative reaction toward the therapist, including rage that the therapist was expecting too much of him. A warded-off but emergent feeling that "recovery was too good for him" was clarified. Frank brought up a past memory of how he, at age 5, had piled toys onto his unwanted 2-year-old brother in an effort to get rid of him. This childhood memory added intensity to his present guilt. Frank was asked to explore the question of how much remorse he needed to feel to reduce his sense of guilt. As Frank worked on this issue, he decided to volunteer his services to teach drowning prevention to schoolchildren, even though the prospect made him tense and anxious. He saw how he could be constructive; this differed from a need to be self-punitive—as in seeking to fail in his current career efforts.

In the termination stage, the plan was to help Frank feel less dependent on the therapist so as to shore up his sense of identity; he feared a relapse after the treatment ended. By the next-to-last session, Frank felt that he would be able to stop at the appointed time, provided that booster visits could be available as needed. Frank and his therapist both agreed to this plan.

TABLE 2–9.   Formulation throughout the course of treatment

Stage of treatment	Steps of configurational analysis
1. Evaluation	1. **Phenomena**
	2. States
	3. Topics and defenses
	4. Identity and relationships
	5. **Integration and treatment planning**
2. Initial support	1. Phenomena
	2. **States**
	3. Topics and defenses
	4. Identity and relationships
	5. Integration and treatment planning
3. Exploration of meanings	1. Phenomena
	2. States
	3. **Topics and defenses**
	4. **Identity and relationships**
	5. Integration and treatment planning
4. Improving coping	1. Phenomena
	2. States
	3. **Topics and defenses**
	4. Identity and relationships
	5. **Integration and treatment planning**
5. Working through	1. Phenomena
	2. States
	3. **Topics and defenses**
	4. **Identity and relationships**
	5. Integration and treatment planning
6. Termination	1. Phenomena
	2. States
	3. Topics and defenses
	4. Identity and relationships
	5. **Integration and treatment planning**

Note.   The steps emphasized in each stage are shown in **bold.**

CONCLUSIONS

Stress response syndromes encompass many diagnoses, the common symptoms of which include excessive intrusive and avoidant symptoms. Although a specific diagnosis may be relevant to some treatment choices, formulation is the ideal route to treatment planning. Configurational analysis is one method of case formulation.

Formulation occurs after evaluation, but the case formulation is revised during every stage of treatment, as more is learned and as initial improvements are observed. Specific steps of configurational analysis are emphasized at specific stages of treatment, as shown in Table 2–9.

CHAPTER 3

Support

Patients often seek professional help weeks or months after a traumatic event because they still have symptoms and an intuitive sense that they are not recovering. Usually these symptoms occur when patients are in an undermodulated state of mind, one characterized by intrusive experiences, dangerous impulses, or a sense of loss of mental control. If so, state stabilization through supportive measures is indicated.

At the biological level, support may include suggestions for restoring proper nutrition and getting more rest; a prescription for medication may be needed in some cases. At the social level, supportive measures may include giving the patient recommendations for time structuring, giving advice to people affiliated with the patient, and guiding the patient into mutual-experience discussion groups. At the psychological level, supportive measures involve establishing a therapeutic relationship while carefully listening to the story of the stressor event and communicating possible treatment plans. The patient gains hope for recovery after perceiving the therapist's empathy and expertise and during discussions of potential therapeutic benefits.

BIOLOGICAL SUPPORT

Sleep disruption is one of the most frequent symptoms in stress response syndromes, although it is not specific to this disorder. Restoration of unmedicated normal sleep is the best biological support, albeit not easily achieved. Patients should be taught how to develop good sleeping patterns. Such advice may include instruction on how to alter their habitual time structure to allow for naps, earlier bedtimes, and uninterrupted sleep insofar as it is logistically feasible. By contrast, some insomnia symptoms are helped by restricting extra sleep time (Krakow et al. 2001). In addition, relaxation techniques may reduce the frequency and/or duration of hyperarousals and tense states of mind. If nightmares have recurrent themes, their content should be reviewed and counteracted in psychotherapy. Sedatives for sleep are usually not indicated because of the potential for overuse, habituation, and possible addiction. However, some selective serotonin reuptake inhibitor antidepressants are sedating and may, if indicated, be taken at bedtime.

Hyperarousal burns sugar, and stress may lead to fatigue and weight loss or even gain in the instance of insulin insensitivity. Encouragement to eat regular meals and avoid strict diets may be part of sound nutritional advice. Recommendations against excessive eating of high-calorie comfort foods when distressed might be offered. The stressed person is less inclined to prepare balanced meals, and adequate nutritional advice should take this into account.

Stress can affect many neurotransmitters, the autonomic nervous system, and hormonal functions, as well as their interactive processes. Changes in electrochemistry affect neural networks that connect the limbic, frontal cortical, basal ganglia, and hypothalamic structures. Disturbances in the physiology of these networks can disrupt arousal control (as manifested in increased frequency of startle reactions and irritability) and diminish the person's capacity to regulate alarm reactions (as in fright responses). The amygdala may alter danger-recognition set points; the hippocampus may alter memory-encoding properties; and the medial prefrontal cortex may alter its ability to establish or reduce (desensitize) associational connections.

LeDoux (1996) and LeDoux and Gorman (2001) reviewed the known anatomic pathways for the development of conditioned fear in animals, pathways most likely the same as those in humans. Stimuli are relayed from the external environment through the sensory pathways of the thalamus and cortex to the lateral nucleus of the amygdala. In this nucleus, a conditioned stimulus and an unconditioned stimulus are integrated. On subsequent exposure to the conditioned stimulus, signals that enter the lateral nucleus are given an especially fearful meaning. The lateral nucleus activates the central nucleus of the amygdala, which then activates brain-stem areas, producing various fear-type reactions.

Connections with the periaqueductal gray region control freezing- or immobility-type responses. Connections with the lateral hypothalamus control autonomic nervous system functions that probably produce a range of responses in humans, from heart-pounding arousal to fainting. Connections with the paraventricular hypothalamus control endocrine responses.

LeDoux (2001) suggests a mode of biological support by emphasizing the social psychology of active coping, on the grounds that in the state of actively doing something well, information transmission can be diverted to the basal nucleus of the amygdala rather than mostly to the central nucleus. From the basal nucleus, connections extend to the striatum and motoric circuits. The more a person engages in active coping, whether it be coping with a specific fear-arousing stimulus or coping with some other aspect of life, the less vulnerable that person is to experiencing a protracted passive fear reaction. The active coping need not be stress-event-targeted; instead, the point is to increase actions related to self-efficacy.

Chemical imbalances may also occur as a part of stress response syndromes. A prominent catecholamine altered in reactions to stress is dopamine. Dopamine is concentrated in the norepinephrine-rich areas of the brain. These brain regions are connected to the emotional arousal–regulating functions of the amygdala as well as to the rest of the limbic system and hormonal systems from the hypothalamus to the pituitary gland and outwards to other bodily systems. Dopamine and serotonin may be involved in heightening biological propensities for hyperarousal and hypervigilance. Repeated alarms can lead to fatigue and further dysregulation of cognitive-emotional functioning (Southwick et al. 1993). Trauma-induced alterations in this neural chemistry could lead to either fight–flight arousals or states of relative immobilization.

Long-standing biological changes occur in chronic posttraumatic stress disorder (PTSD). These may generally affect both immunological and stress response systems. For example, in combat veterans with chronic PTSD, central nervous system levels of norepinephrine were found to be higher than those in healthy men; these levels positively correlated with the severity of current PTSD symptoms (Geracioti et al. 2001). These biological changes link to psychological ones with probable intercausality; that is, adrenergic hypervigilance and arousal can promote intrusive thinking via activation of the brain substrates of these functions. Social triggers of psychological associations that activate neural substrates of intrusive thinking can also promote reactive release of adrenergic substances. Treatment that can alter excesses or deficiencies in any area of linked intercausalities is likely to benefit all elements in the linkage.

As mentioned, the hypothalamic-pituitary-adrenal axis is involved with stress, anxiety, and depression, and a variety of hyper- or hypocortisone level responses may occur. It is speculated that in extreme instances high sustained cortisol can temporarily or possibly affect permanently the hippocampus with it important memory processing functions (Yehuda 2001). Sensitization of the hypothalamic-pituitary-adrenal axis may also lead to hyperarousal after severe stressor events, but because of complex interactions hyposensitization could occur.

Biological support should include careful attention to substances used in attempts at self-medication to reduce alarm or fatigue. Patients often increase their consumption of alcohol or heroin as a sedative, nicotine or cocaine as a stimulant, and marijuana or St. John's Wort as a mood-altering agent. Patients should be advised against such self-medication in favor of physician-prescribed regimens. Also, the clinician should review all of the patient's prescription drugs from doctors and dentists to ensure that excessive amounts, interactions, or unwarranted continuations are avoided.

Antianxiety and affect-dampening medications are sometimes prescribed to prevent extremes of desperate agitation, emotional flooding, and racing, disorganized thoughts. Transient use of such medications is sometimes effective as a way of reducing explosive entry into extremely undermodulated states. These agents can be used in a single dose or as a very short-term approach when critically needed; however, regular, extended use may lead to dependence or addiction. In most instances, antianxiety agents such as benzodiazepines should be avoided. Instead, patients in whom anxiety and depression are both present should be prescribed a selective serotonin reuptake inhibitor (SSRI) with antianxiety effects. For other patients, β-blockers may be useful as a temporary way to reduce extreme physical signs of anxiety.

Sometimes a therapist will encounter a patient who has already been on a benzodiazepine-type drug for more than 2 weeks. Cessation of the medication may be indicated. Abrupt withdrawal is seldom indicated, however. The best course is gradual withdrawal depending on the type of drug, dosage, and length of use (Benzer et al. 1995). With heavy drug use, a formal withdrawal procedure may be indicated and may include in-hospital treatment and physiological monitoring. In such instances, other medications may be used to support equilibrium during a difficult passage. With lighter use, the dosage of the benzodiazepine-type drug can be tapered off, with an interval of a few days at each taper, and the use of 10%–15% less dosage at each increment.

Benzodiazepine withdrawal symptoms include anxious states of mind, insomnia, depression, depersonalization, headache, nausea, abdominal pain, palpitations, chest pain, visual hallucinations, paranoid thinking, and other experiences similar to those of alcohol and sedative withdrawal syndromes (Miller 1990). If the patient was taking a longer acting benzodiazepine, then the withdrawal symptoms may be worse on days 3 through 10 after the medication is terminated. Symptoms may take several weeks to attenuate.

An interesting question concerns whether and when to use sedation during the actual occurrence of stressor events. Usually this question will arise during medical care. For example, combinations of anxiolytics–sedatives and painkillers are already routinely used as conscious sedation during medical procedures such as colonoscopy and coronary angiography. These combinations have memory-reducing effects as well. In one small study of 21 survivors of cardiac arrest, long-acting sedation after resuscitation predicted a favorable outcome, assessed in terms of fewer PTSD symptoms (Ladwig et al. 1999).

SSRIs, tricyclic antidepressants, and monoamine oxidase inhibitors have all been used in the treatment of PTSD with some reported success. The SSRIs have been shown to be superior to placebo in several well-designed studies (Brady et al. 2000; Davidson et al. 2001a, 2001b; Marshall et al. 2001). At this writing, the U.S. Food and Drug Administration has approved sertraline (an SSRI) for the treatment of PTSD, and paroxetine, another SSRI, is, at the time of this writing, likely to win approval.

In some patients, recurrent schizophrenic episodes may be precipitated by stressful life events. At such times, prescribing of antipsychotic medications (or adjustments in dosage) may be indicated.

Patients with stress response syndromes can become suicidal. Clinicians should be alert to the possibility of prescribed medication's being used for that purpose. Contractual agreements with patients to not attempt suicide sometimes bolster adaptive coping efforts and morale. Whenever it can be realistically enhanced, hope is a good medicine. Caution, however, should be used in regard to the volumes and types of medications prescribed.

SOCIAL SUPPORT

Persons who are exposed to traumatic events often experience themselves as overwhelmed. Social support is extremely valuable. Those who provide this support often need reassurance and advice. The following principles are helpful in this regard.

1. The patient may need to be transiently protected from excessive stimulation. Time structuring following a disaster should emphasize short-range activities that foster a sense of safety, control, and social connection.
2. Provide the patient with opportunities for communication. Discussing the event with others may be useful in differentiating realistic and unrealistic interpretations. Debriefing support groups can also be helpful soon after shared stressor events such as an earthquake, a building

explosion, or an airplane crash. Mutual-help groups can be extremely valuable even long after an event such as the death of a child, a cancer diagnosis, or heart surgery.

3. Providing timelines for dose-by-dose coping can restore a sense of personal efficacy to a bewildered or overwhelmed patient. Even a Scarlett O'Hara approach of "I'll think of that tomorrow" can be adaptive if not prolonged.

4. Activities should be interspersed with periods of respite. It is important for the person to feel that it is all right to rest or to change activities for a period of restoration. Activities that restore a sense of social connection and foster positive states of mind are valuable. A variety of systems for relaxation are available that may be useful in this regard. These range from deep-breathing exercises to systematic muscular relaxation or other somatic slow-down modalities such as Tai Chi, yoga, and meditation. Music, art, dance, reading, television, walking, or sports may provide restorative episodes that, for a time, allow the person to put aside unresolved stressor topics.

5. Giving the person something to do in the role of helping others may help restore a sense of worth, competence, and self-esteem. Otherwise, consider a transient reduction in caretaking responsibilities.

6. The more a person has been traumatized, the longer it will take for his or her symptoms to subside. This reality may conflict with the expectation in some work environments that the traumatized person will return to his or her usual functional level within a few weeks. The workplace provides sustaining interest and social support; the person should not be isolated from it, but neither should he or she be required to meet excessively high expectations regarding recovery.

7. Children who see repetitious film clips of a disaster on TV may believe that the depicted event is really happening over and over again. They need adult explanations to reassure them that they are safe and that the dangerous conditions are over.

8. Because sleep disruption is common in stress response syndromes, the patient may associate efforts to sleep with episodes of unpleasant imagery. Adjustments in the environment to provide an increased sense of safety can be helpful. These might include leaving lights on or sleeping with a pet. Children might be allowed to sleep with a parent temporarily, even though that may not be the usual domestic arrangement. In extreme cases, telling the patient that a companion will stay awake and watch over him or her during sleep can encourage rest.

9. A person who has experienced a recent trauma may be more at risk for having an accident while driving or operating machinery. For these reasons, keeping the patient from driving unnecessarily or doing hazard-

ous work tasks may be advisable for a time. This must be done tactfully so as to avoid fostering self-concepts of incompetence.

10. Often, immediately after a traumatic event, the person's relatives and friends will cluster around and want to know what happened, and the victim will recount the story again and again. Although for some individuals this is valuable, for others it is not and can even be maladaptive. Later in time, when companions may be tired of hearing about the traumatic experience, the victim may still feel the need to review what happened. The therapist can advise family and friends that merely being with and listening to the patient fulfills a useful function. Companions do not have to offer solutions, directives, probes, or unsolicited interpretations to see themselves as helpful.

PSYCHOLOGICAL SUPPORT

Telling the Story of the Stressor Event

Telling the story of the stressor event to a competent therapist is an important initial support event because it occurs in a context of relative security and calm, unlike the patient's previous experiences of telling the story to potentially critical persons such as police, other victims, or relatives and friends. A feature of this security warrants mention: the therapist needs to be aware of his or her own reactions to hearing stories of trauma. The realities disclosed can be horrible; the therapist can be repelled or fascinated and can become emotionally drained or preoccupied. Personal memories of a traumatic nature may also be triggered, thereby causing the therapist to experience a variety of countertransference reactions.

Telling the story involves more than recounting reality; it includes inner responses as well. These responses consist of fantasies that the person had during as well as after the stressor event, and sometimes before. A patient may say, "I knew that this would happen to me one day, and I expected it would be like..." Differentiating the reality from the fantasy aspect of the story will be important in every aspect of treatment; for very distraught patients, the difference between fantasy and reality need not be totally interpreted in the support stage.

Telling the story includes reactions to associations to a series of cascading events. That is, although a criminal assault takes center stage as THE STORY, in actuality this event leads to a cascade of other stressor events such as encounters with law enforcement officers, hospital personnel, insurance providers, lawyers, and relatives or friends, who may have seemed hostile, self-interested, or unsympathetic.

Therapists often see patients who have not fully developed the components of stories into accurate temporal sequences. Patients seldom have a complete view of the cause-and-effect sequences that are involved in a chain of events. Clarification of these sequences merely starts in this stage of treatment; it will continue in later stages of the psychotherapy, especially those involving the exploration of meanings and the working through of conflictual themes.

Providing Information and Structuring Tasks

Some patients are in such a state of overload that they can only absorb small amounts of new information. But many, although they are novices to the traumas of life, are able to learn about stress responses and develop coping capacities. The therapist can provide information in a series of short statements. For some patients, supplemental materials can be provided, such as bibliotherapies or videocassettes. Such resources include books such as *Coping With Trauma: A Guide of Self Understanding* (Allen 1999), *Life After Trauma: A Workbook for Healing* (Rosenbloom and Williams 1999), and *Post Traumatic Stress Disorder Sourcebook: A Guide to Recovery, Health and Growth* (Schiralde 2000). For disaster victims, certain Internet resources can be useful, such as the Web sites of the Federal Emergency Management Agency (www.fema.gov), the Red Cross (www.redcross.org), and local protective resource institutions.

A plethora of things to do or contemplate floods every victim of a traumatic event. Confusion can result. In such instances, but not in a way that fosters dependency, the therapist can help in structuring tasks. Topics for contemplation can be prioritized when the time comes for making necessary decisions. Actions can be ordered by efficacy as well as urgency: *efficacy* refers to actions that can be accomplished readily and can also enhance a sense of capability. Writing down what is said is often valuable, given that memory fluctuations occur under stress.

Stressor events can be traumatic because they carry a lot of important and possibly dire implications, and because they constitute a shock to previous self-assessments: the person is not in as much control as he or she had assumed. The realization about not being in full control of the situation can lead to an extreme and overgeneralized response, such as "I cannot control anything." Such a response is more likely to persist in a person who before the stressor event had a fear-evoking attitude most of the time. This overgeneralized response can also be latent if it has been replaced by an overt attitude of self-efficacy. For individuals who, subsequent to their traumatic experience, engage in repeated expressions of "I cannot control anything," realistic corrections are indicated to reduce catastrophic overgeneralization (Bandura 1977; Beck 1976). Replacement suggestions can be made, such as

"There are things I can control, but these other things are beyond my control."

Establishing a Therapeutic Alliance

As mentioned, hearing others' stories about their traumatic experiences can evoke empathic reactions of horror, terror, disgust, or revulsion in the clinician. Although such reactions are normal, they can increase the patient's tension. In addition, some patients test therapists by attempting to provoke reactions such as fear ("I cannot help such a patient"), hopelessness ("No one could ever cope with that"), or withdrawal ("I cannot take in such extreme emotions"). For these reasons, therapists should be alert to their countertransference reactions. Other common countertransference responses involve the therapist's unconsciously taking on the role of victim and feeling fear and hopelessness, or taking on the role of an aggressor and feeling like a sadist who forces the patient to relive memories of bad times.

Wilson (1994) and Wilson and Lindy (1989) have compiled a useful list of frequently occurring countertransference reactions reported by therapists who treat trauma patients (Table 3–1). By recognizing their vulnerability to such reactions, therapist and other social support persons can minimize the potential of communicating negative feedback to the patient and foster restoration of the therapeutic alliance.

Under strain, some people regress to withdrawn, desperate, or excessively anxious attachment patterns. Unfortunately, individuals prone to desperate forms of contact-seeking behave in ways that alienate those who might otherwise help them. By recognizing their own countertransference reactions, therapists can avoid alienating patients and can help them to reduce provocative or unresponsive stances with others.

Establishing appointments, a diagnosis, and a formulation can be quite reassuring to patients. Conveying facts can reduce secondary anxieties. Some people, for example, presume that intrusive symptoms represent an unusually lowered control over their mental contents and interpersonal emotional expressions—they fear they are losing their minds. The therapist can allay such fears by providing patients with accurate information about the prevalence of symptoms, such as intrusions after a serious life event, as well as the usual course of improvement. Patients can be told that they need not focus their attention continually on the intrusive memories, ideas, and feelings. Putting such topics temporarily out of mind can restore equilibrium. It does not mean that they will be either forgotten or avoided forever.

Such temporary reprieves from focusing on stressor topics can be fostered through "dosing" of emotion. The therapist can help prioritize which

TABLE 3–1.   Common countertransference themes in posttraumatic therapy

Emotional countertransference issues

Anger at the source of victimization

Anger at client because of the intensity of affect

Anger at society for failure to help victim

Fear of affective intensity in client

Fear of personal vulnerability and potential for victimization

Anxiety over ability to help the victim

Guilt over being exempted and not suffering

Empathic sadness and grief reactions upon hearing the trauma story

Feelings of dread, horror, disgust, shame, and revulsion upon hearing the trauma
   story

Numbing of responsiveness in response to psychic overloading induced by the
   trauma story

Deliberate avoidance of the trauma story which may be conscious or unconscious

Cognitive countertransference and interpersonal strategies

Belief that a "therapeutic blank screen" approach is an appropriate stance (false
   neutrality)

Overidentification with the victim

Overcommitment to helping the victim

Excessive belief in personal responsibility to shoulder burden of therapy

Ideological and clinical disillusionment produced by the trauma story

Conception of self as rescuer, savior, gifted healer (narcissism)

Form image of client as weak, pitiful, and not capable of overcoming
   traumatization

Belief that medication will alleviate affective intensity and give the therapist
   control

Belief that posttraumatic stress disorder does not exist

Belief that stress symptoms are premorbid in origin (were present to same degree
   before the stressor event)

Source.   Reprinted from Wilson JP: *Trauma, Transformation, and Healing: An Integrative Approach to Theory, Research, and Post-Traumatic Therapy.* New York, Brunner/Mazel, 1989, p. 205. Used with permission.

topics require current consideration and which topics could be contemplated later. Attention to positive emotional memories or future opportunities can be encouraged as well.

A theme for some patients is that of feeling less attractive to others when in posttraumatic states of mind. These patients cringe because they believe others will see them as cowards, weaklings, malingerers, or as boring or ugly companions. The therapist can provide realistic reassurance by letting the patient know that this is a common stress response. This information can partially restore a rational perspective.

An important part of formulation in this early stage of support is the therapist's and the patient's observations of change in interpersonal patterns that are a consequence of the trauma. In many instances, the stressor event will have led to altered states of mind, which can cause a disruption in the sense of self as part of a community. Adaptation is fostered by fellowship, group belonging, and appropriate levels of help. Conversely, maladaptation may result if the patient heightens his or her dependency on unreliable sources of support, angrily rejects support because it falls short of magically erasing the trauma, or hides out to avoid potentially embarrassing social interactions. These interpersonal tendencies are diagrammed in Figure 3–1.

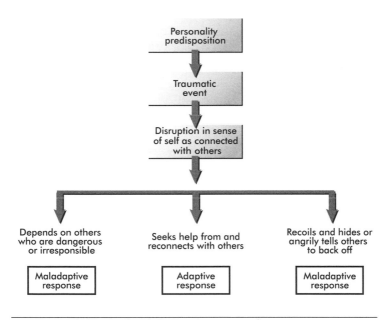

FIGURE 3–1. Adaptive and maladaptive interpersonal responses to trauma.

Establishing a commitment to care by presenting a plan for what will be done provides both empathy for the patient's level of current distress and hope for change. Such initial support can lead to a sharp reduction in symptoms. The patient can then move rapidly toward exploring meanings, improving coping, and working through in the ensuing stages of psychotherapy.

CASE EXAMPLES

The first case example below illustrates ways a therapist can help a patient find support in a social context and avoid unnecessary medication. The second example illustrates the therapeutic support given to a couple experiencing marital disruption after the death of a child.

Maria

Maria, a 40-year-old widow, sought a consultation 1 week after the death of her husband of 20 years. He had had terminal cancer, and she had expected his death for some months. Disrupted sleep and feelings of agitation and shame were her chief complaints.

Maria's overmodulated state of mind caused her to conduct her life in a ritualized and numb manner. Only when attempting to sleep did she experience undermodulated states of repetitive worry about her behavior. Her main topic of concern, associated with these states of agitation and shame, was why she had remained stoic and tearless at the funeral. It seemed that the other people who attended the service had tears at some point; therefore, they must think that she did not love her husband. She described this concern with intensity but she restrained her personal emotions. Her demeanor conveyed an urgency that the therapist do something to ease her mind. This role had been taken on by her primary care physician; he had given her a prescription for nighttime sedation that she had not yet filled.

The psychotherapist began with support and waited to see if any further interventions were indicated. She told Maria that she would be available to help her grieve if that were needed, but she had some information now that might be useful. She said that it seemed to her that Maria expected to grieve at the same rate as others as at the funeral. This was not a reasonable expectation, because Maria cared deeply for her husband and was more involved with him than were the other people—he was still mentally a large part of her everyday life. The therapist went on to say that people who cared deeply needed a long time to mourn; they sometimes had a period of emotional numbing until it felt safe to start grieving with more feelings of sadness, anger, remorse, or whatever else might come up. Dry eyes at or after the funeral was not an indication that Maria did not care.

Maria asked questions about this intervention and gradually seemed to understand it. She felt relieved of her guilt about not crying, and of her shame at the imagined accusations of others. She also spoke of guilt reactions about her thoughts of being relieved that her husband's last days of suffering as well as her tension were ended by his death. The therapist listened sympathetically in a manner that socialized as acceptable such feelings of relief. She told Maria that different feelings about her loss would likely occur as time passed; there was emotional memory and life-restoring work yet to take place.

The urgency to do something was reduced. Maria indicated a change in her dysfunctional belief about not crying at her husband's funeral. The therapist suggested that Maria try not to use sleeping medication; instead, she should allow herself unusually long times for sleep to take place, including naps. Another consultation time was scheduled to consider what would be helpful to Maria in her mourning process, which was expected to take place over weeks and months rather than days.

Alex and Andrea

Alex and Andrea were tormented by a terrible event, the death of their only child. To make matters worse, they were experiencing a fracture in their marriage during this time of intense need for mutual support. Their son had fallen while playing on a cliff and had died after a neurosurgical attempt to save his life. Both parents felt depressed and lost interest in sexual relations. The couple came together for consultation 6 months after the event.

As in the case of Maria but extending for months, Alex exhibited denial and numbing but experienced intrusive thoughts and pangs of feeling about the loss. His symptoms met the criteria for PTSD. Andrea experienced continual pining for her lost son and other symptoms meeting the criteria for major depressive disorder. Andrea wanted to talk about memories of their son with Alex, but he avoided these discussions because they increased his sense of overpowering loss. Andrea felt isolated, rejected, and angry at Alex's avoidance of these topics.

The situation was serious, with both husband and wife moderately to severely disrupted in their social functioning. Feeling unsupported, each considered divorce. The therapist expressed sympathy for both of them. He explained that it was normal for them to have different phases of response and also different styles of coping with this most stressful of all traumatic events. He advised individual psychotherapy with different therapists.

The therapist told Andrea and Alex that with their permission, he would remain in touch with the individual therapists, and he would be available for conjoint sessions with them. The individual therapies would focus on their loss, and the conjoint therapy would focus on their marital interactions. In the meantime, he offered a practical suggestion: The couple could not usefully never talk about their son, nor could they expect to both benefit from talking a great deal about him. Could they, however, just for now, agree to a kind of time limit for such a conversation to take place? Andrea and Alex discussed this idea and came up with a "5 minutes per dose" agreement. They both seemed relieved and closer as a consequence of having decided on this strategy, and they accepted referrals for individual work with different therapists.

CONCLUSIONS

Understanding a patient's personal response to trauma can help reduce their secondary fears, those fears that are based on the erroneous beliefs about what is normal or abnormal, current or permanent, hopeful or hopeless, acceptable or stigmatized. The cases of Maria, Andrea, and Alex illustrated how patients can be expected to go through phases of stress response in a variety of ways. It is important that the therapist provides each patient adequate education and helps him or her to have realistic expectations.

Patient support is examined across biopsychosocial approaches. Case formulation leads to a selection of which combinations of approaches could be used in an individual treatment. Because people vary in their response to traumatic events, the degree and kind of support would also vary.

Whereas most patients need the most support early in treatment, there are instances where a patient needs fewer supportive interventions early in treatment and more supportive interventions later on. There are several reasons why some patients need this later support. One reason is that the patient might fear experiencing emotional consequences of remembering the traumatic event. With exploration of meanings, the next stage of treatment to be discussed, the therapist may come to realize that the patient is frozen in a denial numbing state. By increasing support at this later point, the patient may feel safer and set aside the control processes that have led to his or her denial.

Another reason a patient may need more rather than less support during a later stage of treatment is that the cascade of life events that may follow a single stressor episode can be overwhelming. For example, after death of a child, parents may divorce due to feelings of estrangement. The loss of a spouse, the legal hassles, and the lapses in engagement by mutual friends may all compound the patient's sense of disaster. Increased support measures will be indicated.

Some treatment approaches may result in increased emotional distress and symptom exacerbations; increased later support will again be needed.

Support restores the patient's hope and reduces the tendency to give up in the face of stress; it also prepares the patient to gradually take on increased levels of responsibility, thereby contributing to a more positive sense of self.

CHAPTER 4

Exploration of Meanings

By this stage of the therapy, the patient will have told many stories related to the stressor event. Indeed, some patients will have recovered enough that the therapist can proceed to termination. For many patients, however, an exploration of the stressor's meanings will be both necessary and emotionally difficult. The presence of the clinician as a compassionate and empathic person who is trained to think logically helps this process.

Exploring meanings exposes discrepancies between the world as it was experienced before the stressor and the world as interpreted after the event. This mismatch evokes strong feelings. The therapist sanctions expression of these emotions as part of establishing a therapeutic alliance. The therapist helps the patient to handle potentially overwhelming feelings by dividing his or her expression of these feelings into tolerable dose-by-dose experiences. Establishing a sense of safety allows the patient to explore meanings that may have been warded off to prevent entry into undermodulated emotional states. The patient is helped to remain in working rather than overwhelming expressive states.

A brief conversation from a psychotherapy session will serve to illustrate what is meant by sanctioning emotion. In this session, the patient was describing a recent and sudden rejection by her lover at a time when she was already under stress from losing her job.

Patient: *(Sobs)* I just can't handle it.
Therapist: To have him turn away from you just then must have been very difficult.
Patient: *(Slight derisive laugh)* It's just…I don't understand.
Therapist: Yes. *(The therapist indicates that he understands her pain and confusion and is there to support her; he encourages her to say more.)*
Patient: I don't understand why people are that way. Oh dear, I'm going to cry again.
Therapist: That's okay, you probably have some crying to do. *(Sanctions emotion.)*

When the clinician discovers a block that prevents the patient from contemplating the meaning of the serious events to the self, he or she can help the patient by stating that such blocks are self-protective ways to avoid being emotionally overwhelmed. The therapist then encourages the patient to share the experience in a safe way; this is done by representing him- or herself as a person who will not be overwhelmed by contemplating the implications of illness, injury, or loss. The clinician thus helps the patient to learn by identification.

A REVIEW OF PHASES OF RESPONSE

A generalized prototype of phases of response to a trauma was summarized earlier in Figure 2–1. It often is helpful to educate a patient about such phases. This process sanctions both time on and off the topics that generate intense negative affects.

The outcry phase is usually over by the time the patient is ready to explore meanings. However, patients fear recurrence of the horror of this phase. They may reflect in therapy on questions that occurred to them in the immediate aftermath of the stressor event, such as "Why me?" and "How will I ever be happy again?" Exclamatory statements made during the outcry phase—such as "I am to blame for everything that happened!" and "I can never recover from this, all is lost!"—need to be reviewed. The therapist then helps the patient separate realistic from unrealistic appraisals of what the stressor means to the self.

In phases of denial, attention may be focused on improving a sense of safety, because it is a sense of dangerous vulnerability that makes denial necessary. Sometimes the therapist must confront inhibitions that are maladaptively prolonged, a topic covered in Chapter 5. The clinician may also need to interpret the views and feelings that were warded off by extreme defenses such as blanket avoidance.

In the intrusive phase, the therapist aims toward reducing the sense of shock and alarm that may occur with each recollection of the traumatic memory or each perception of a stimulus that is associated with the trauma. This often involves telling and restructuring the story of the disastrous events as the therapist helps the patient to understand cause-and-effect sequences and to differentiate facts from fantasy. By placing each concept associated with a trauma within a time frame and sequence, the therapist facilitates a sense of reality and integration of what has happened into a personal life story with a hopeful future.

Magical conjectures about what might have caused the catastrophic event can be counteracted by clear, lucid, and more rational reappraisals. The therapist may also bolster the patient's self-esteem by emphasizing the patient's positive traits and attributes. The goal is to return the patient to a sense of competence and worth.

In the working-through phase, further desensitization of emotional associations and the restructuring of beliefs occurs as larger frameworks of meaning are explored. The person deals with conflicts reactivated from the past by the recent stress. The topics may include memories and fantasies of earlier traumas. The self-concepts may involve activation of degraded self-schemas that were latent before the trauma.

By encouraging contemplation of the ideas and implications to self associated with the stressor event, the therapist hopes to gradually increase the patient's capacity to tolerate emotions. Conceptions of the self as worthless, incompetent, bad, shamed, guilty, or weak are challenged. New, adaptive practices are examined for efficacy. This process of contemplation and practicing new behavior leads to a change in cognitive maps (this phase will be discussed further in Chapter 6).

In the completion phase, the patient's future functional capacity and resilience to future stressors are discussed. After a stressor illness, such as a heart attack for example, it may be useful to distinguish between realistic and unrealistic expectations regarding the patient's future degree of ability and disability. Coping ability may be enhanced by preparing a plan for what to do and how to react if similar stressor events recur.

TOPICS OF CONCERN

Formulation and reformulation during this exploratory state of therapy will have identified topics of concern. The patient will still be associating the stressor event and specific responses to it with the more general network of meanings in his or her life; this will include memories and fantasies from the past. Because of this work of association, some aspects of remembering and appraising a recent trauma will be revised.

Meanings may change as the patient tells and retells the story of the trauma. Therapists should not be surprised by this; it is common. In addition, the quality of memories may change. Repeating a memory may decrease image intensity and affective alarms; this usually indicates a positive change. Signs of increasing image intensity and distress may indicate that deeper expression is taking place, but they can also mean that the memory is unresolved. Unresolved memories present topics for more work. Relevant signs of resolved versus unresolved memories are summarized in Table 4–1.

TABLE 4–1.   Memory of the stressor event: unresolved or resolved

Unresolved	Resolved
1. Excessively imagistic and quasi-real	1. Less vivid recollection
2. Nonvolitional repetitions	2. Voluntary recollection
3. Emotionally evocative (alarms and emotional pangs)	3. Less sharp emotional activation
4. Difficult to dispel	4. Can shift attention away from memory
5. Unclear if real or unreal	5. Clearer sense of what is memory and what is fantasy
6. Hard to relate to identity	6. An aspect of identity

CASE EXAMPLE

Francisco

Francisco presented for treatment because of firm and, as it turned out, quite astute recommendations from his primary care physician and a specialist in endocrinology. For some months, he had been so apathetic in pursuit of his career as a tax and payroll accountant that the family income had fallen into dire straits. Francisco no longer took any satisfaction in work, and he stopped making the evening house calls that had been his specialty in tax work for couples.

Francisco no longer enjoyed bowling with his family and friends, nor was he taking pleasure in his other social activities. He had no libido and no work drive, yet he did not meet the criteria for any depressive disorder. His primary care physician referred him to an internal medicine specialist for a workup for possible hypothyroidism.

When medical examinations and tests came back normal, Francisco was referred to the university specialist in endocrinology. His endocrinology tests also came back normal, so a careful history of his symptoms was again taken. The history revealed that Francisco's problems of low energy and apathetic behavior had begun after he had been robbed at knifepoint one evening on his way to a tax consultation.

Because Francisco's symptoms began after a trauma and were not explained by any medical diagnosis, the endocrinologist referred him to the university stress research clinic to explore possible causes of his condition. Francisco was skeptical but cooperative. No formulation was arrived at during his evaluations; however, there was a clear temporal connection between symptom onset and the assault. A time limit of 10 to 12 sessions was set. Because support was not indicated for Francisco, treatment began with exploration of meanings.

Francisco began in a passive-aggressive mode. He said little. That led the therapist to use a question-and-answer format. Francisco's nonverbal communication expressed an attitude that indicated the therapist's questioning would be futile. Nonetheless, the therapist took an expanded case history. The family history indicated some friction between Francisco and his wife, but this could well have been secondary to his changed demeanor and their financial difficulties. The history of the assault and its aftermath was reviewed in detail. After four sessions, the therapist was still unclear on how to formulate the case.

Francisco spoke of the assault without defensive signs and without emotion. He described his current avoidance of being out during the evening as a rational choice; he had been irrational to feel so invulnerable before the assault, but now he knew better. He wished to relate better with his wife, but what could he do when he felt tired all the time? He was not depressed, angry, or ashamed and even seemed resigned to his condition staying as it was.

The therapist went back and asked Francisco to redescribe every detail of the assault episode: the shape of the man, the sound of his voice, the knife, what he had thought at each moment, and what he felt when the man took his watch and wallet and left, after making a menacing swipe toward him as if to demonstrate what would happen if Francisco called for help. Francisco gave mechanical details and rather colorless associations that provided no further information on which the therapist could base a formulation. If Francisco's condition was in fact associated with the assault, the therapist reasoned, the man must be in extreme denial. Deciding to explore this possibility, the therapist became confrontative. As if speaking on Francisco's behalf, he said, with emotion, "That crook would have made me so angry!" Similarly, he exclaimed at another point, "That would have terrified me!" Francisco reacted neutrally to these emotional remarks as if the roles were reversed—he was the calm therapist and the therapist was an emotionally distraught client. The hour ended with the therapist feeling quite pessimistic about reaching any explanation for Francisco's problems.

Francisco came for the next session displaying emotional states of mind for the first time. He reported a nightmare in which there had been a burglar in his basement: Francisco armed himself with a hatchet, went down the cellar stairs, and towered over a weak man—Francisco was about to chop him into pieces. The therapist said, "Imagine how the burglar felt." "Afraid," said Francisco, tentatively.

Francisco had felt very frightened during and after the real assault, but he had masked it with a cloak of such inertia and withdrawal that the connection between his apathetic condition and the trauma had been lost. With the link made, he then dealt primarily with anger as a response. He verbally lost his temper with his wife, kicked her during sleep, and also kicked the wall.

Francisco began to speak of his own fright. He recalled how afraid he had been during the assault; he had been paralyzed with terror, thinking that the knife might strike his guts. Even though he was emotionally distressed during the series of interviews, he progressed to the improving coping and working-through stages (these are addressed in Chapters 5 and 6, respectively). Later in therapy, Francisco gradually resumed other life functions. As a result of having tempered both his preassault omnipotent invulnerability and his postassault hypervulnerability, he was able to achieve a restored sense of safety.

UPGRADING FORMULATIONS

As a consequence of having fully explored the meanings to a patient of a recent stressor event, the clinician will have more ingredients for a formulation of the case than he or she had at the time of the initial evaluations. These ingredients can now receive further consideration. Formulation will be addressed, as before, by using the configurational analysis groupings of information into states of mind, topics of concern (because they are important and unresolved), and beliefs arranged into schematizations that organize identity and relationships.

States

After a stressor event, people often experience a dilemma: although they want to master the stressor by confronting it, confrontation can lead to feared states. They attempt to circumvent this dilemma by avoiding confrontation; however, although this strategy may offer escape from horrors, it does not restore their desired state of calm equilibrium.

As a way of exploring such wish/fear dilemmas, states of mind can be organized according to the configuration shown in Figure 4–1. The configuration's four quadrants consist of a desired state, a dreaded state, a problematic compromise state, and a protective compromise state. One of the compromise states is less adaptive because it contains vexing symptoms such as anxiety states; the other looks more adaptive because it attenuates symptoms such as anxiety, but it does not represent mastery. It is a protective compromise, and because it is only quasi-adaptive—it is an uneasy resting place for patients who may still have symptoms such as avoidance and numbing.

Figure 4–1 illustrates this aspect of formulation, a common configuration of states after a very traumatic event. The figure depicts the degree of emotional control within these four states: well-modulated emotion in

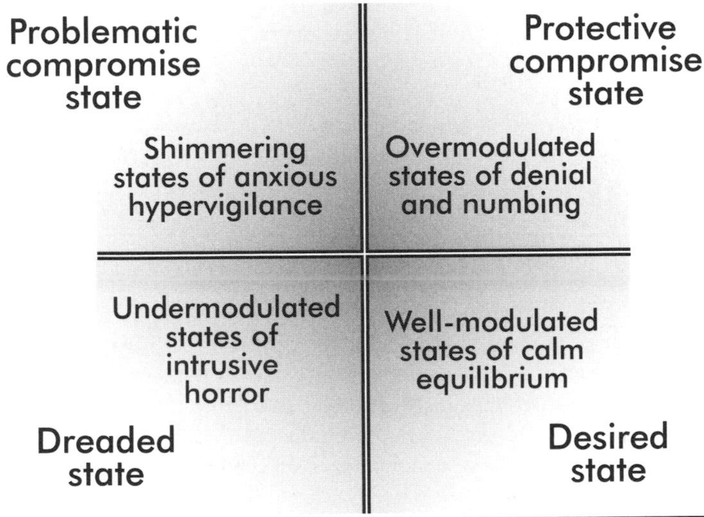

Problematic compromise state	Protective compromise state
Shimmering states of anxious hypervigilance	Overmodulated states of denial and numbing
Undermodulated states of intrusive horror	Well-modulated states of calm equilibrium
Dreaded state	**Desired state**

FIGURE 4–1.   Desired, dreaded, and compromise states of mind after trauma.

desired states, undermodulated emotion in dreaded states, overmodulated emotion in protective compromise states, and shimmering of emotion in problematic compromise states. Shimmering includes contradictory signs such as tightening of the mouth, looking sad in the eyes, and disavowing emotions verbally.

Topics

Because a vivid emotional contemplation of unresolved topics tends to lead patients into dreaded states, defensive efforts are made. These efforts are often attempts to control emotion. Such control processes may shift topics or alter the way ideas within a key topic are represented and associated. In problematic states, some elaborations of ideas and some expressions of feelings may occur, but others are also warded off, as when tears come to a person's eyes and are then blinked away while the person gives a false-appearing smile. This give and take-back effect produces the shimmering appearance of many problematic states.

More extensive emotional control processes may produce protective states. The key unresolved stressor topics may be avoided—or, if expressed, the person may shift to alternate self-views, thereby fostering a sense that the event did not occur in the center of his or her personal life. Projective mechanisms may also be used, wherein the dreaded emotions are attributed to someone else.

For these reasons, in upgrading formulations, it will be useful to link key topic events both to state-shifting patterns or cycles and to repetitive inhibition, distortion, or projection patterns.

Self-Relations

The important, unresolved, and emotional topics that stem from traumatic experiences will often contain conflicts about roles for self and others. Further formulation of identity and relationship problems is usually indicated. Such formulation is especially important in patients who have dissociative experiences. In such inferences, it is helpful to examine variations of self-other beliefs in different states of mind.

Each state of mind that is recurrent in a person is organized by an active or dominant schema of self. A self-schema is an organized compendium, a patterned aggregation of elements. It functions as a package of unconscious associated meanings about the self. Each self-schema is a constellation of subordinate components such as body images, roles, scripts for relating to others, symbols, values, fears, desires, constraints, intentions, expectations, action plans, and styles of self-control.

Self-schematization, as shown in Figure 4–2, is a nested hierarchy of beliefs: each supraordinate unit combines many subordinate bits of information. The self-knowledge assembled in such schematizations is both reality based and fantasy based. The information is both procedural and declarative, explicit and implicit. The time frames are current, past, and projections into the future. Much of the schematized knowledge is unconscious; however, many derivatives can be represented for conscious self-observation.

Trauma often activates dormant or latent aspects of self-schematization. Stronger self-schemas are weakened, and latent, weak self-schemas are primed. A change in the person's conscious sense of identity can result.

This concept bears repetition because it is so important in understanding multiple states of mind in a person. A self-schema, one of several within a repertoire, can be active or inactive in affecting current thought, emotion, perception, and action. An active self-schema leads to a style of thinking, communicating, and acting. Traumas can alter the relative activity of self-schemas. Associations about the trauma can prime a self-schema that was relatively inactive before the stressor event and cause it to become a very active organizer of the person's subsequent experiences. The activated schema may contain exaggerated beliefs of personal inadequacy, which can then interfere with optimum adaptation.

Supraordinate Schemas

As mentioned, a conscious sense of identity is based on derivatives of self-schemas. Because multiple self-schemas are activated, many different iden-

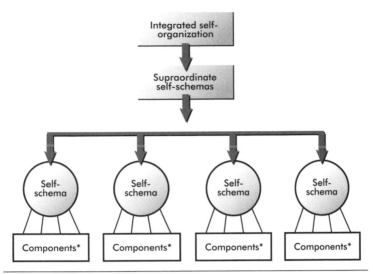

FIGURE 4–2. Self-schematization.

*Components of self-schemas include body image, roles of self, habitual desires, values, emotional response style, habitual self-regulatory style, scripts of habitual action sequences, future intentions and plans, and key memories of self.

tity experiences may result. The more the person has coherent linkages of multiple self-schemas into supraordinate schemas, the more continuous will be that person's sense of identity over time. The less the integration before the trauma, the greater the possibility for chaotic identity experiences in the posttraumatic period.

Role Relationship Models

Identity experiences are associatively primed and supported by current relationship experiences. Associations of self with other can be captured as a role relationship model. Such a model forms a cognitive map of the attributes, characteristics, and scripts of potential transactions of self and other. Scripts include future plans of self-intentions to move toward desired possible future identities and away from dreaded ones.

In associative processing, the possible meanings of a trauma are compared with each organized schematization of self in a relationship. Some people fear that usually latent schemas of personal vulnerability may be activated because of associative linkages of the actual vulnerability of self with the stressor events. If these dreaded schemas have not been previously attenuated by supraordinate schemas that can contain and diminish them, a regressive decompensation may occur. For example, an adult who has recently endured a traumatic experience may become especially distressed if the roles of a similar childhood trauma have never been mastered. Conversely, if those roles were mastered, the adult may adapt resiliently.

Role relationship models can be formulated for each salient state of mind (desired, dreaded, problematic, and protective). Doing so is valuable because the models are predictive of possible transference reactions that may complicate the therapeutic alliance. Such reactions are based on both positive and negative expectations. An illustration of an expanded configuration related to the states already discussed is shown in Figure 4–3.

As shown in Figure 4–3, the most dreaded state is one of intrusive horror. In terms of a negative transference expectation, the patient sees him- or herself as a helpless victim and the therapist as a powerful aggressor who mercilessly requires the patient to recount the story of the traumatic event, repeatedly subjecting the patient to an unwanted reliving of memory. The expectation is that the patient will express all of his or her vulnerabilities experienced during the trauma, will then be attacked by the therapist for not expressing his or her memories better or fully enough, and will experience terror at having to endlessly repeat a story that is so disturbing. Although this is not a rational expectation of a therapy situation, the traumatic repetition can be an unconscious expectation. For example, a victim of a rape assault may unconsciously expect that the therapy, in and of itself, will somehow represent a repetition of the rape—in effect, penetrating the patient's mind by forcing him or her to talk about some of the physical acts.

A less intense negative transference expectation can occur in the problematic compromise state, one of anxious hypervigilance. In this state, the patient may self-identify as a needy victim who is making demands for help but expects that the therapist will be an inexpert or inconstant helper who will fail to meet his or her needs. The result is mistrust with the potential for rage because the help provided did not meet the patient's needs. As a defense, the person can move into a denial–numbing state that represents a kind of resistance to a therapy state; it is a protective compromise that does not have the anxiety, rage, or terror of the dreaded or problematic compromise states.

As seen in the upper right quadrant of Figure 4–3, the patient represents him- or herself as an apathetic victim encouraged by the therapist. The therapist is viewed as having characteristics of untrustworthiness. To ward off emotion, the therapist's attempt to encourage retelling the trauma story must itself be warded off. The resultant countertransference is that the therapist may be left feeling useless or helpless to do the necessary work.

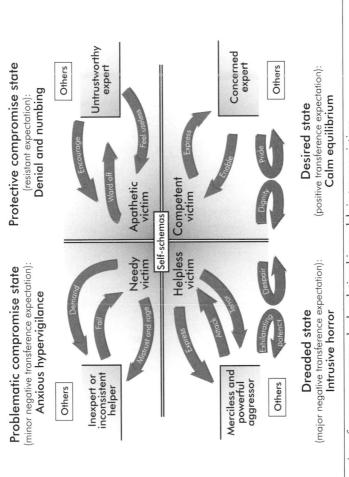

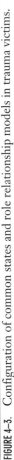

FIGURE 4-3. Configuration of common states and role relationship models in trauma victims.

The desired state can also lead to positive transference expectations, possibly excessive ones. The patient may assume a false state of calm equilibrium even though he or she has not yet worked through the trauma event. The self-role is that of competent victim working with a concerned expert who is enabling the victim to tell his or her trauma story. The person feels a restored sense of dignity, and the therapist feels a countertransference reaction of pride in the success of their work. This can be an excessive positive transference expectation if the work that has been done is not actually progressive in mastering the trauma, and if there is an unrealistic view on the part of the patient that excessively idealizes the therapy situation and the therapist.

For many patients, notational systems and multifaceted formulations such as those shown in Figure 4–3 will not be necessary. However, for patients in whom reactions to stressor events are combined with preexisting personality problems, these more complex formulations are valuable.

CONCLUSIONS

Exploring meanings in the supportive context of therapy helps the patient to think about what has been hard to face. As these difficult topics are communicated, the clinician revises his or her formulation and makes further plans for what needs to be accomplished in treatment. The next stage of treatment covers improving the coping capacity of the patient, therefore as part of reformulation, it is important to consider the patient's defensive resistances and core beliefs about identity and relationships.

CHAPTER 5

Improving Coping

After a reformulation based on explored meanings, the therapist can plan how to help a patient improve his or her coping strategies and capacities. These plans often include interpreting attitudes that lead to unnecessary avoidance of unresolved topics. The therapist encourages the patient to confront current crises more directly in tolerable doses and emphasizes making new decisions for handling stressful situations.

Such confrontations can lead to increased experiences of negative affect and general tension, but these can be reduced by the hope provided from the supportive situation. As already mentioned, common stress management procedures can also be helpful: relaxation exercises, stretching, meditation, breathing, massage, yoga, biofeedback, and systematic slow body movement like Tai Chi or Feldenkrais. The secondary messages of endorsing such stress-reduction methods are 1) take time for self-restoration, and 2) avoid self-calming and self-stimulative attempts that rely on street drugs, alcohol, nicotine, risk taking, and promiscuity.

The memory of a stressor event may still evoke shock. This sense of alarming emotional arousal may be partially due to a gross mismatch between trauma perceptions and prior expectations. The following case example illustrates this kind of mismatch.

CASE EXAMPLE

Teresa

Teresa had been physically assaulted by her husband. Before the attack, he had exhibited episodes of rage, but during the assault, she had seen for the first time an expression of destructive hatred on his face. Her previous view of him had been one of a loving husband who lost his temper a bit when frustrated; it had never included a concept of his wanting to annihilate her. When Teresa saw her husband's monstrous rage, she was shocked and overwhelmed. She began to experience a recurring memory image of his villainous face; it was an intrusive repetition of her shocking realization. Part of the shock was that she had no way to handle such an unexpected and dangerous situation.

Now, with Teresa in therapy, her husband seemed sincerely apologetic, solicitous, and seductive. She stayed in the relationship and continued to live with him while denying the repetitive possibility of his assaults. The therapist identified Teresa's belief that her husband would never hit her again as unrealistic. It would be important, he said, both to prevent repetitions and to also be ready with a plan should another assault appear imminent. The therapist told Teresa that he believed that their repeated discussions about her relationship with her husband would help her to face the reality of her husband's various and extreme states of mind. By contemplating the totality of the situation, she would be further enabled to form realistic goals for changing her marital relationship, including whether or not she wanted it to continue.

With Teresa, the therapist planned to be alert for possible emergent dysfunctional beliefs such as, "I must be with him to be a worthwhile person," "I must never express my anger or I'll be rejected," or "If I don't fill all his needs I am a total failure." If these beliefs emerged, the therapist planned to clarify and compare them with alternative and more adaptive role concepts. Also, should another assault occur, Teresa would be prepared with her own assertive plan of what to do and whom to call for help. Because Teresa self-owned such plans, the therapist expected her to experience fewer entries into a dreaded state of mind.

CONSCIOUS AND UNCONSCIOUS CONTROL OF EMOTION

Teresa sought to avoid the topic of a possible repetition of her husband's dangerous rage attack. The therapist knew that Teresa's coping could be improved if she were able to replace her pathogenic defensiveness (excessive inhibition of the topic) with more adaptive conscious controls of thought. Such defensive avoidance operations are common in stress-induced disorders.

In a study of 66 patients with posttraumatic stress disorder (Horowitz et al. 1980), the most common methods of avoiding personal emotional meanings of the stressor event were the following:

1. Excessively inhibiting associational connections (found in 69% of the patients)
2. Excessively switching attitudes to avoid emotion (64%)
3. Distorting reality to avoid deflations of self-esteem (41%)

Each of these avoidant strategies may be usefully counteracted by the therapist to work on stress-related topics and devise plans for how to handle specific situations. Some techniques for use with people who habitually inhibit ideas, avoid emotion, and distort reality for self-enhancement are presented in Tables 5–1, 5–2, and 5–3, respectively.

TABLE 5–1.   Avoidance and counteraction with people who habitually inhibit ideas

Defensive avoidance of the patient	Counteraction of the therapist
Is inattentive and gives only sketchy or disjunctive details about the event.	Encourage talk on the topic and provide specific words. Ask for details. Then construct cause-and-effect sequences by clarifying time and sequence.
Inhibits specific subtopics.	Confront the avoided topic through gradual clarifications.
Short-circuits to maladaptive conclusions and decisions to avoid emotion.	Keep the topic open, emphasize step-by-step decision making, and recheck plans for effectiveness potential.
Makes misinterpretations on the basis of past stereotypes of self and other without attempting new and realistic appraisals.	Interpret what is realistically likely and differentiate that from what is most dreaded and what is ideally desired. Differentiate reality from fantasy. Clarify intentions and motives. Distinguish beliefs about possible futures from beliefs about the past.

REDUCING FEARS OF REPETITION

Many patients are inordinately afraid of situations in which a repetition of their trauma is realistically unlikely. Phobias may result. Exposure techniques are sometimes useful for reducing an oversensitivity to intense fear states and for bolstering self-confidence.

Exposure may involve either memory evocation or real situations. However, when asked to evoke memories, patients may be fearful because they expect that such repetition will lead to retraumatization. This fear is a legitimate one. Patients may also dread entering real situations. For this

TABLE 5–2.   Avoidance and counteraction with people who habitually avoid emotion

Defensive avoidance of the patient	Counteraction of the therapist
Gives excessively detailed story about peripheral rather than emotionally central concepts about unresolved stressor topics.	Ask for central and personal meaning.
Avoids speaking of feelings.	Interpret the most likely linkage of emotional meanings to expressed ideas. Focus some attention on metaphors, images, and bodily felt reactions.
Juggles opposing sets of meanings back and forth.	Hold discussions on one subtopic.
Dyselaborates (takes back) what was said.	Interpret defensive shifting and what it conceals.
Endlessly ruminates without reaching any decisions on how to cope with a situation.	Interpret reasons for procrastination. Encourage action planning and model the process of examining the comparative efficacy of alternative plans.

reason, the therapist must have a clear rationale for exposing the patient to threatening stimuli and must explain that rationale to the patient.

The effects of exposure should be evaluated. The desired outcome is not to reexperience terror but rather to decrease the intensity and negativity of affective arousals. The goals are desensitization, a reduction in overgeneralization, and a progression from terror to calm. In the past, techniques known as "abreaction and catharsis" sometimes retraumatized patients if they were not conducted in a way that increased rather than decreased a sense of calm and self-control.

Exposure with the goal of facilitating desensitization of conditioned fear responses can involve memory, fantasy, guided visual imagery, role-playing, and/or returning to environments associated with the stressor. The clinician selects what he or she feels is the best approach for accomplishing the desired desensitization of triggers to emotional alarm reactions and undermodulated, dreaded states of mind. Once again, the goal is to achieve as much calm during the exposure as possible; with the repetition of heightened calm, the patient's emotional equilibrium will be restored.

The rationale for exposure involves learning theory in the context of how

TABLE 5–3. Avoidance and counteraction with people who distort reality for self-enhancement

Defensive avoidance of the patient	Counteraction of the therapist
Focuses on praise and blame for actions during stressor event and is deceitful about what happened.	Avoid being provoked into either praising or blaming; do not accuse of lying.
Denies information that deflates self-concepts.	Use tactful timing and wording to counteract distortions of meaning.
Is evasive or misdirective in giving information about who did what to whom to protect self from shame and guilt.	Consistently redefine meanings and encourage realistic appraisals while bolstering against shame.
Uses grandiosity as a coping attitude.	Cautiously deflate grandiose meanings while emphasizing realistic skills and capacities.
Excessively quick forgiveness of self for culpability.	Support patient while working toward an appropriate sense of what really happened. Help patient plan for realistic acts of remorse; encourage pride in taking responsibility.

emotional habituation occurs. Progressive familiarity with previously frightening stimuli can increase calm if the repeated exposure occurs within an associational network of other stimuli that represent capability, support, safety, and optimism. The person's increased calm decreases the strength of the conditioned associational linkages between the stress-related stimuli and fear arousal. That is why it is important to assess whether a restoration of equilibrium occurs as a consequence of exposure techniques. If it does not, the alarm reactions may be further conditioned and the person retraumatized.

Simple rating scales can be employed to measure whether reductions in distress are indeed occurring. Use of a 10-point scale with "the most distress you could possibly experience" rated as 10, and "no distress whatsoever" rated as 0, can be helpful in obtaining patient reports of inner experiences during exposures. The patient rates the experience with each repetition. Seeing reductions in distress can reinforce hope in the outcome of the exposure techniques.

In addition, exposure techniques can help the person reorganize his or her cognitive map of how the traumatic event relates to the self. A cognitive map is a conceptual generalization that can include major beliefs and event expectations as well as person schematizations such as role-relationship models. Exposure can alter the weight given to dire expectations, decreasing a sense of threat. In addition, the exposure repetitions facilitate emotional information processing. The therapist encourages the patient to distinguish how the current stimuli are similar or different from traumas in the past and also fosters a heightened sense of self-efficacy (Foa and Meadows 1997; Foa and Rothbaum 1998; Harvey and Bryant 1999).

The most common exposure technique involves memory rather than a therapist-supported return to the trauma site. The patient is asked to remember the experience of the traumatic event in an individual or group therapy setting. Remembering can range from recounting a portion of the story to more intense reliving. The therapist starts the patient at the low emotional dose end of this range. Another common technique of exposure uses imagery. The therapist suggests specific scenarios to visualize. During such imaginal exposure, gradations from mild to intense are used; the suggested images gradually move from less to more distressing experiences.

In vivo exposure, in contrast to imaginal exposure, involves direct confrontation of the situation and site of the trauma. The patient returns, with a supportive companion, to the place or type of place where the trauma occurred. Again, one can use a graduated range of avoided or phobic situations. The person first confronts a place or situation likely to induce only mild anxiety. He or she then gradually confronts situations that might arouse more distress. This approach provides a learning experience that with appropriate support can help the person to feel progressively calmer in situations and places that were previously avoided.

It is sometimes helpful to teach the patient how to release tension that may build up during exposure procedures. Muscle relaxation, breath control, postural changes from guarded to more relaxed positions, and rehearsal of what to say to the self are useful techniques for this purpose. Self-talk can include such positive phrases as "I can handle this," "I've done it before and I can do it again," "No fear," or "I am not alone."

After exposure, it is important to review the experience. This includes assessing associations and clarifying any dysfunctional beliefs. The therapist should repeatedly contrast dysfunctional beliefs with more adaptive alternative beliefs.

Because exposure can lead to an increase rather than a decrease of intense and negative emotions, it is again important to emphasize a dose-by-dose approach in discussions with the patient. This means teaching the patient both how to start and how to stop paying attention to a threatening topic. At first the therapist presents alternative topics for contemplation to encourage consciously mediated (i.e., deliberate) attentional shifts. The therapist may use role-playing techniques to show the patient both how to remember and how to change the topic of contemplation. Methods for attention control without the presence of the therapist can then be taught.

DISSOCIATION

During and after very traumatic experiences, dissociative processes may complicate adaptive cognitive-emotional work. Dissociative processes can lead to depersonalization and derealization. They can segregate emotional memories or schemas into relatively nonassociated networks of meaning (Foa and Hearst-Ikeda 1996; Zatzick et al. 1994). For this reason, some clinicians have used hypnotic techniques to 1) locate the dissociative memories and 2) reduce the schematic segregations by suggesting connections between otherwise encapsulated sets of ideas and feelings (Spiegel and Classen 1995). Hypnotic techniques engage attention in a highly focused and circumscribed way.

Because of the context of suggestion in which hypnosis is induced, it may, at the same time, reduce the patient's sense of responsibility for thinking and feeling. This is sometimes counterproductive. Suggestions for active and adaptive coping attitudes can be offered during hypnosis by the experienced therapist. Most clinicians, however, tackle dissociation without use of hypnosis, and it probably should not be used by clinicians who are not highly experienced in its methods and knowledgeable about its advantages and disadvantages.

PHASE ORIENTATION

Orienting treatment plans to the phase of the patient's responses may be quite valuable. Most patients will oscillate in their states of mind; they will have some states with intensely emotional intrusive recollections and some states with emotional numbing and ideational avoidance. A few patients, however, may still show signs of either more extreme denial or more extreme intrusion (rather than an oscillation with attenuated signs of both). For such patients, different sets of techniques may be considered. In extreme denial circumstances, the therapist can interpret attitudes that have made total avoidance a defensive necessity and can suggest how using less avoidance can still be safe. In extreme intrusive circumstances, the therapist can structure suggested activities to allow the patient to increase control over behavioral sequences, emphasize benevolent environments, and reduce energy-consuming demands. Some phase-oriented interventions are shown in Table 5–4.

IMPROVING DECISION-MAKING CAPACITIES

With reduction of global defensiveness and heightening of selective conscious control, the patient's sense of restored self-efficacy can be enhanced

TABLE 5–4.   Phase-oriented interventions to improve coping

Patient phases	Therapist interventions
Extreme denial phase	Increase sense of safety.
	Change attitudes that make excessive controls seem necessary.
	Suggest attention to unresolved topics.
	Suggest expressive activities such as role-playing, artwork, joining a support group.
	Interpret how and why emotion is being stifled.
	Reconstruct story of the trauma and aftermath to prime memory and associations.
Extreme intrusive phase	Structure time and information for patient.
	Encourage activities associated with capability even if they are not direct stress-coping activities.
	Reduce external demands and stimuli.
	Recommend rest.
	Provide models that the patient can use for personal roles.
	Clarify and educate about stressor and stress responses.
	Suppress emotional thinking—for example, with meditation, relaxation, soothing music.
	Evoke other emotions—for example, emphasize positive memories, benevolent environments, hopeful futures.
	Desensitize stimuli that cause alarm reactions.

by helping the patient take increased levels of responsibility for rational decision making. Such decisions include whether to, when to, and how to remember traumatic events; how to cope with present situations; and how to handle changed relationships with others. They also include developing skills for setting priorities, for determining what to do when, and for deciding which goals come first, second, and third.

Once plans are derived from decisions, repetition is important. Resolution of contradictions will be the hardest task. With further development of self-reflective consciousness, the patient can link antitheses into rational explanations and make choices for resolving dilemmas. In this process, the therapist can help by providing a framework for reducing the clash between attitudes. For example, a patient may be oscillating between guilt over harming or not protecting others and rage at people who did not protect the patient and others. The patient may blame other people as a way of reducing his or her own guilt or shame. Instead of activating rage to stifle guilt, the patient can be helped to acknowledge both the blaming and the personal remorse. The thought that either oneself or others are totally to blame is a form of extremist thinking and is irrational. The self is neither totally guilty nor totally revenge preoccupied. This middle ground represents a rational softening of extreme attitudes.

The therapist can also provide a route through conundrums and dilemmas that recur in thought and interpersonal situations. If the patient comes to self-own such a route and to repeat it in trains of thought, he or she will know what to do with recurring preoccupations on unresolved topics. A symbol system can be established whereby the person can say to him- or herself, "I have thought this through before and decided that...so I do not have to dwell on it in my present unproductive state of mind."

For victims of stressor events, coping with guilt and shame is sometimes harder than coping with fear and anger. This is especially true if during the event the person caused harm to others, failed to protect others from suffering more injury than he or she suffered, or felt glad to survive at their expense. In such instances, the therapist should not echo the blanket reassurances often used to soothe trauma victims; reality-guilt is sometimes present. Fantasy-guilt, however, is more prevalent. Both are psychological realities within the mind of the survivor and need to be confronted as such.

Coping with guilt can be addressed as an unresolved topic of concern, with its own polyphonic complexities. Suppose, for example, that a patient has a repetitive intrusive thought, "I should have died like the others." This thought may be associated with self-punitive or even suicidal impulses or potentials. If so, the therapist can ask the patient how much and what kind of remorse would be required to complete his or her guilt response. Self-punishment is irrational, unproductive, and harmful to family, friends, and colleagues. Restitution, as in good works to help others, is often a more adaptive way to expiate guilt. Another way of coping with unresolved topics is to use the conventional "meat and potatoes" psychotherapy technique of helping the patient review cause-and-effect sequences so as to differentiate reality beliefs from fantasy beliefs.

It is helpful for the therapist to share with the patient his or her observations about how the patient's coping capacity has incrementally improved, from "back then" until "now." The therapist can also focus on how the patient's improved coping with the sequelae of the recent stressor event might extend into the future by increasing the patient's general resilience, courage, and stamina. The enhancement of self-confidence that results will reduce vulnerability to states of anxiety and depression and will prepare the patient to undertake tasks of further working through of unresolved and intensely emotional topics.

CONCLUSIONS

Patients often have difficulties coping with the memories of a trauma and the continuing crises that stem from the stressful event. Therapists can help these patients improve their coping capacity by 1) countering avoidances that are no longer necessary in the present situation of improved safety, 2) reducing unrealistic fears of a repetition of the trauma, 3) decreasing startle and alarm reactions, and by 4) improving reasoning about what did happen and what can now happen to improve the situation. The therapist can help patients find new ways to make decisions about conundrums and dilemmas, and to discover new skills for self-efficacy. The therapist can bolster the patient's self-esteem by pointing out where progress has already been made in their improved coping skills.

CHAPTER 6

Working Through

Complex, conflicted, and dilemma-ridden topics are especially difficult to resolve without expert help. Reaching a resolution of such themes takes time and usually requires modification of beliefs, attitudes, and schemas of self and affiliation. To help a patient make such revisions and reschematizations, interpretive and conceptual reconstructive work is required. This is especially true when working with the deeper levels of intervention, those that concern irrational beliefs, maladaptive identity and relationship concepts, and plans involving fantasies about the future.

These deeper levels of intervention relate to the surface levels that were discussed as part of the earlier stages of treatment. In the earlier stages, communications in therapy focused on 1) topics of the stressor event and personal responses, 2) choices of how to cope with stressful new situations that are part of the trauma sequelae, and 3) avoidance. These earlier stages of treatment also focused on 4) the occurrence of dreaded states of mind and how to reduce their potential for maladaptive effects. From this level of state analysis and recognition of unresolved topics, it is sometimes valuable to go deeper into what is less consciously apparent—that is, to 5) unrealistic expectations and irrational beliefs, 6) the relationship of current problems to prestressor potentials for maladaptive interpersonal patterns as well as prestressor problems of identity and self-organization, and 7) conflicted and fantasy-based planning for possible futures of the self.

This list of seven levels of possible attention and intervention by the therapist addresses the choices that need to be made on the basis of the therapist's up-to-date case formulation. In treating stress response syndromes, the common principle is to go no deeper than necessary; the therapy should go only as deep as is needed to restore equilibrium and to help the patient achieve his or her optimum functioning. In patients who require a more extensive working-through process, an interaction of meanings and feelings stemming from the stressor event with preexisting meanings stemming from personality-formative experiences is often present. Expert judgment is needed to decide how far to go in interpreting the interaction of stressor-related and preexisting personality problems.

In part, this clinical judgment is simplified by experimenting with the temporal focus that helps to achieve the most progress in each therapy session. The choices are to focus on current outside situations, on current in-therapy situations, on the past, or on some combination of any two or all three of these foci. The relationship of these temporal foci to the levels of topical focus is shown in Table 6–1.

Table 6–1 may be used as a way to consider what the therapist is doing with a patient in treatment. Where is the therapist currently focusing his or her interventions? Why? What are the consequences of focusing, for example, on the past origins of irrational beliefs rather than on differentiating current realistic and unrealistic appraisals? Does it help to link a specific pattern to the patient's realistic or unrealistic expectations of the therapy process?

All of these topical and temporal foci for therapist attention and intervention can be used in the exploration of any area that requires further working through. As mentioned, the themes that require the most extensive work usually are entangled with personality. Some of the most common themes of this type include the following:

- Excessive fear of future victimization
- Enduring and irrational shame over vulnerability or incompetence
- Unusually intense anger and impulses for revenge
- Extreme sensitivity to guilt
- Low thresholds for despair with expectations of being abandoned

EXCESSIVE FEAR OF FUTURE VICTIMIZATION

The nervous system's development of conditioned fear responses occurred in the course of evolution as a way to protect the organism from experiencing a repetition of assaults and noxious situations. The fundamental nature of such conditioning means that the organism carries a primal tendency to fear certain futures. Beyond this reflexive functioning, humans add ideational–emotional projections into various possible futures. Some people develop an excessive fear of victimization as a conse-

TABLE 6–1. Levels of intervention

Level	Topical focus	Temporal focus		
		Current	Now in therapy	Past
1	Stressor event and personal responses	Plans of how to prepare for future stressor events	Expectations of treatment	Relevant previous stress events
2	Choices of how to cope with stress	Conflicting plans of how to cope with consequences of recent stressor event	Choice of therapy focus	Long-standing goals and dilemmas
3	Avoidance of challenges	Defensive avoidances and distortions	Encourage work on important topics	History of self-impairing avoidances
4	Dreaded states of mind	Triggers to entry into symptomatic states	States of therapeutic work (and nonwork)	Habitual dreaded states
5	Irrational beliefs	Differentiation of reality-based from fantasy-based appraisals	Reasonable expectations versus fantasized hopes	Origin of unrealistic expectations
6	Maladaptive interpersonal patterns	Interpersonal problems and degradations of identity	Difference between transference and therapeutic alliance	Relation of current problems to past patterns
7	Life plans	Opportunities for adaptive change	Harmonizing conflicted beliefs	Development of intentions

quence of having experienced a severe stressor event.

As discussed in preceding chapters, desensitization procedures can help reduce conditioned fear responses and thus phobias of future repetitions of a recent disaster. Intellectually, however, both patients and therapists know that there is always a chance of a stressor event's being repeated; among the many possibilities, another person may be murdered, one could be raped again, or another car accident might occur. The process of working through consists of realistically appraising and differentiating between the repetition of fantasy-based and reality-based fears.

The most potent fantasy-based fears are ones involving an irrational view that one caused the recent trauma oneself. For example, a person who has a fantasy about shooting fellow students in his or her school can magically interpret his or her vindictive thoughts as the reason why a similar tragedy took place, in reality, in a different school. People with magical thinking often expect and fear that their traumatic experiences will be repeated.

Excessive fear of future victimization may also develop if the recent trauma has become entangled with associations to past traumas. For example, the traumatic event may have been a car accident in which the patient, who was a passenger, was injured because of the reckless driving of a friend. In one unresolved topic, the patient might feel like a victim of the reckless friend who was driving the car. The patient may have an important past experience of being a weaker person assaulted by a stronger person. The current injury and its causes may become entangled with a memory of childhood fears of harm at the hands of that stronger person. The patient may then have fears of the future that are based on both the more recent and the more remote memories and schemas of self and other. Any future situation of not being in personal control may be exaggerated into anticipations of being under the control of a stronger and harmful other person.

It is a judgment question as to how much the therapist should explore childhood memories in such situations. Reliving is not necessarily beneficial; it can lead to retraumatization. It is best to start with the current appraisals and to proceed deeper with caution and, as already discussed, only if necessary. Going deeper will also lengthen the time for the patient to be in therapy.

If, before the recent stressor event, a person had debased self-concepts, he or she might use those beliefs as reasons to explain why the trauma occurred; dysfunctional beliefs such as, "I will always be the victim," or "I must deserve to be a victim," may be repeated as internal cognitions or spoken statements. It is important to repeatedly clarify and confront such beliefs. The goal for the patient is to be alert to such assertions to counter them with clear, adaptively positive self-statements. To repeat: the emphasis is on noting, stopping, and counterstating such dysfunctional beliefs. As will be discussed later in this chapter, these beliefs are often associated with preexisting themes of shame and/or guilt.

ENDURING AND IRRATIONAL SHAME OVER VULNERABILITY OR INCOMPETENCE

Recent stressor events can make a person feel ashamed of his or her vulnerability or inability to help others. Some events may socially stigmatize victims and intensify their shame. Wishes to hide away during traumas may also be recalled and appraised as a source of shame. These emotional attitudes are more difficult to resolve when a recent traumatic event activates preexisting roles of the self as weak, deficient, degraded, defective, and negatively exposed by the criticism of others. Shame makes one feel terrible and weak; it can be undone, in part, by activating rage at others.

UNUSUALLY INTENSE ANGER AND IMPULSES FOR REVENGE

Anger at the source of a trauma and a thirst for revenge on the aggressor(s) is also a common conflicted theme; it may serve as a self-strengthening, defensive shift away from shame. Irrational attitudes may hold innocent others as aggressors. For example, rage at a drunken driver can be displaced onto paramedics who arrived to help, but not as quickly as desired. Such rage can activate latent role relationship models with a scenario of self as unfairly hurt, and other as an aggressor or a deliberately unreliable caretaker. As long as most or all blame is directed outward, the anger feels righteous. But blame can shift inward, followed by a sense of guilt at the self for having been too angry and vengeful. The conflict between expressing and stifling hostility is reactivated by rage at the loss, injury, or fright one sustained from the stressor event. The prior vulnerability schemas make normal rage more intense.

Sometimes rage is directed at those who did not suffer as one did. This recognition, that self was damaged more than others, may awaken previously conflicted but relatively latent personal themes of envy. Life seems so unfair that rage may be directed toward oneself as well as others, and suicidal impulses may occur.

Anger reactions take place with high frequency in stress response syndromes (Chemtob et al. 1994). Impulsive violence may also occur. Therapists should be careful to not take this hostility as a personal affront. Countertransference reactions to anger conflicts are common; a therapist may be treated with unjustified hostility by an easily angered patient and become annoyed in response. For these reasons, it is vital that therapists be alert to their own ire. It is also wise to avoid therapist overload from seeing too many such patients.

The problem of the patient displacing rage onto inappropriate targets should be identified. The therapist can help the patient learn procedures for alert control of hostile impulses (Bryant 2000). Work on communicating reasonably well-modulated anger is indicated. The patient's focus of attention can be directed toward the onset of his or her first feelings of frustration; expression and reappraisal should occur early before tension and hostility have escalated to high levels.

When dealing with intense angry themes, it is often valuable to follow the pathway of questions such as, "Who is to blame?" Some anger stems from an externalization of blame from self to others. Sometimes anger is generated by shifting blame from some prior aggressor to an innocent person who is in the immediate environment. The level of hostility may be reduced by repeating concepts that counteract the projective distortions in the appraisal of blame. When general irritability is present, potential methods of self-soothing can be discussed and adaptive approaches (jogging, hot baths, naps, music, reading) can be differentiated from maladaptive ones (drugs, cigarettes, alcohol, starting fights, high-speed driving).

EXTREME SENSITIVITY TO GUILT

Guilt, real or imagined, about actions or failures to act during the trauma may reactivate relevant guilty themes developed in childhood. In *survivor guilt*, the person may believe, consciously or unconsciously, that he or she survived or suffered less at another person's expense. In *separation guilt*, the person may believe that he or she abandoned the victims who died: to avoid blame or make amends, the person magically believes that he or she must join in death or suffering with the more damaged victims. In *omnipotent responsibility and guilt*, the person may assume exaggerated responsibility for aspects of the disaster or the suffering of others. Such guilt themes inhibit the person from moving forward to embrace life after the trauma. In severe cases, when traumatization exacerbates previous guilt themes, people may act out in self-destructive ways. In such instances, the therapist may need to work on enhancing the patient's sense of deserving to heal.

LOW THRESHOLDS FOR DESPAIR WITH EXPECTATIONS OF BEING ABANDONED

Low despair thresholds precipitate entry into states of despair and depression when events lead to loss. Loss may include loss of bodily functions and loss of comfort, as in chronic postaccident pain syndromes. In the case of loss of loved ones or of body parts, a mourning process usually takes place in which the grief relatively resolves. Nevertheless, unresolved grief is more likely in people who have been too frightened of sadness to allow grief work to occur. Depression is more likely in those with biological or psychological vulnerabilities to such states; people with preexisting insecure attachment personality configurations may be especially vulnerable.

TECHNIQUE

For each conflicted theme, repeated attention is given to how the person uses generalizations from past experiences to envision and rehearse for the future. The therapist continually counters unrealistic future expectations with more realistic ones. In addition, rational cause-and-effect sequences are repeatedly presented to substitute for dysfunctional and irrational beliefs about what caused the stressor event. Beliefs from the past that lead to dysfunctional beliefs in the present are clarified to show their lack of current and future validity.

In patients for whom important meanings of the stressor event are clearly linked to dreaded identity concepts and role relationship patterns of the past, the therapist can help by first clarifying the link and then challenging the expectation that past beliefs must dictate expectations of the future. The therapist should reinforce realistic beliefs so that the patient can act to avert victimization, relinquish revenge plans, express remorse, tolerate separations, and live life without annihilation of self.

The following case examples are presented to clarify how linking interventions can be used to maintain a focus on working through an unresolved topic related to a current stressor event. Linking interventions clarify how current concerns may relate to the past, how topics connect, or how inside-of-the-therapy topics relate to outside-of-the-therapy ones.

CASE EXAMPLE

Sally

Sally, a young woman in her early 20s, experienced a severe and complex fracture of her femur; she had fallen from a ladder while helping her father paint his house. Sally sustained a partial paralysis caused by nerve damage. Dread, sadness, and hopeless reactions to this impairment led Sally into depressed states. Her overall condition disrupted her plans to accept a teaching position after graduating from college. She felt hopeless and came for therapy with a diagnosis of major depressive disorder and adjustment disorder precipitated by her accident and its sequelae.

One theme activated by Sally's injury was hostility toward her father for not taking adequate care of her. The relevant ideas about the stress event were that her father had given her a rickety, second-class wooden ladder while he used one that was stable and strong, and her awareness of her anger was partially warded off by continued defensive inhibitions when contemplating this topic.

During treatment, Sally showed signs of anger at the therapist because he would not prescribe sleeping pills for her persisting insomnia. Although the therapist was able to see the nonverbal signs of this emotion, the patient was unable to express them verbally. The therapist considered possible statements he might make. He could say, "I think you may be angry with me but are afraid to say so," or he could link the exploration of the transference anger to the father/ladder meanings of the recent stress event. He decided on the latter tactic and said: "I think you may be getting angry with me right now because I am not meeting your need for a sleeping pill, just as you may be angry with your father because you feel he took poor care of you by giving you a rickety stepladder."

This type of wording links the therapy situation to the current stressor. It maintains the focus of treatment on resolving reactions to recent events.

MATCH AND MISMATCH

If emotional equilibrium was present before a severe stressor event, the person was experiencing states of reasonable calm. That calm reflects a match between the current world and the person's expectations. The trauma event produces a current world that does not match the enduring mental schemas that produce expectations. The results of this mismatch are emotional alarms. As modeled in Figure 6–1, the person then is faced with a dual task: schemas have to be revised to accord with aspects of the stressor event that cannot be altered, and the person has to modulate his or her emotional alarms to the point that they are not overwhelming and causing cognitive disruptions.

If, in contrast, contradictory schemas were present *before* a traumatic event, it may be more difficult for the person to reschematize identity and relationship beliefs *after* the event. Because of internal conflicts, defensive avoidances are more likely to have been schematized. That is, the person has already developed habitual ways of avoiding the negative emotions that lead toward dreaded and undermodulated states of mind. These automatic defenses lead to overcontrol after the stressor event. The effect of this overcontrol—inhibition of information processing—in turn results in inadequate reschematization. This model of not working through is presented in Figure 6–2. The goal of therapy is to help the patient work through his or her overcontrol and contradictory interpretations of the traumatic event so that adequate reschematization can occur.

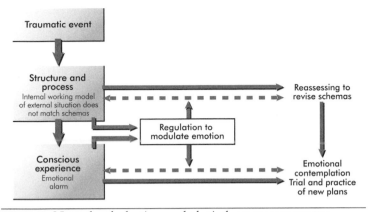

FIGURE 6–1. Normal and adaptive psychological responses to trauma.

Note. *Solid lines* indicate facilitory regulatory processes that advance information processing. *Broken lines* indicate inhibitory or information-distorting regulatory processes that impede information processing.

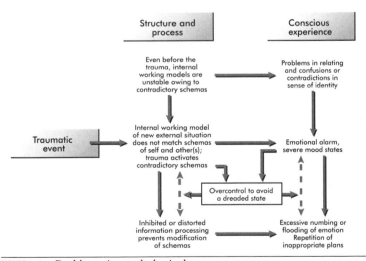

FIGURE 6–2. Problematic psychological responses to trauma.

Note. *Solid lines* indicate facilitory regulatory processes that advance information processing. *Broken lines* indicate inhibitory or information-distorting regulatory processes that impede information processing.

CASE EXAMPLE

Francesca

Francesca was pulled into a park at knifepoint and forced to submit to intercourse on threat of being stabbed. The rapist held the blade to her throat and in a foul, frightening, and painful manner, he violated her. He made a final threat to her life, and left. After an interval during which she felt numb, the memory returned to plague her through nightmares and intrusive images during the day. Francesca was diagnosed months later as having posttraumatic stress disorder (PTSD) and major depressive disorder, both precipitated by the rape trauma.

In the postevent entanglement of meaning structures, the concept "rape" was joined by association to an erotic daydream that was present before the event. In this daydream, a strong, handsome man seduces her by being very forward and nonverbal. In this masturbation fantasy, Francesca was both an attractive and sensual woman and one who was too pure and virtuous to be the instigator of erotic overtures. The strong man, inflamed to fervor by recognition of her beauty, was the one who was responsible for removing her veil of virtuous forbearance. In the safe container of Francesca's daydream, the blame was his; she was the weak person and could experience erotic excitement without guilt.

After the rape, Francesca misinterpreted her recurrent daydream. She viewed it as her "wanting to be raped," and because of this, she felt partly responsible for the assault. She reappraised her own failure to scream for fear of being stabbed as being too compliant. In this way, Francesca activated a degraded and debased self-concept that could be reinforced by social circumstance, such as a police officer or friend asking, "Why didn't you call for help?"

The magical aspects of Francesca's thinking led her to an inappropriate connection between the memory of the real rape and the rape fantasy. Francesca's subsequent association of her traumatic experience to the erotic daydream led to self-blame and hence to shame, guilt, and a dangerous lowering of self-esteem. In working through the stress response syndrome that was set in motion by the rape, it was necessary to repeatedly disentangle the real rape from the erotic fantasy. Francesca needed to realize quite clearly that 1) the real rape was a vicious assault upon her person; 2) the rape was not really linked in causality to her fantasy; 3) the fantasy itself was innocent mental play; 4) she was entitled to be furious with the assailant without self-disgust or guilt; 5) she was entitled to develop a sense of herself as an active, strong, and sexual woman; and 6) future sexual encounters of her choice were not to be magically viewed as enactments of the rape trauma.

In her early childhood, Francesca had not been sexually abused, but a male family member had behaved too erotically toward her. Later in adolescence, she felt that wanting to be sexual was itself taboo. For sexual arousal to occur, she used masturbation fantasies of having sex forced upon her so that she would not be responsible. When she associated these fantasies with the actual rape, the linkage reactivated childhood themes of anxiety, shame, and guilt about personal responsibility for transgressions. Thus,

Francesca's preexisting mental structure of meanings, beliefs, memories, and self-other schemas made the traumatic rape even more traumatic, because it was so difficult for her to work through the dreadful memory of her adult experience and her other associated childhood and adolescent memories. The early memories, the adolescent fantasies, and the recent rape were all likely to cast unfortunate shadows on her future adult sexuality.

A traumatic experience evokes a constellation of themes. The themes include prior self-concepts, prior relationships, and prior emotional memories or fantasies. In patients who—like Francesca—have complex themes, an extended and well-supported period of working through to differentiate past and present as well as reality and fantasy is indicated. A focus on future issues of sexuality is also indicated. Such work usually requires a time-unlimited psychotherapy.

In some managed care situations, the length of treatment permitted for such work may be limited. Clear case formulation on the part of the clinician may supply the necessary ingredients to argue for adequate coverage.

CONCLUSIONS

When a traumatic event leads to development of a postevent syndrome, the clinician may discover that information processing stemming from the event has entangled with memories, meanings, schemas, attitudes, and emotional proclivities from the past. In such instances, the clinician will sometimes need to make interventions at a deep level. The advantage of such a technique, when it is appropriate, is that it provides a silver lining to the dark clouds of the syndrome. Not only can the patient be helped to resolve the symptoms of the stress response syndrome, the patient may gain personal strengths and reduce prior personality conflicts.

Surface interventions are appropriate to what is known about causation of problems early in treatment, when formulations include the first reports and observations available. Middle-level interventions occur as the clinician learns more about the patient and evaluates the progress of the case. Deep interventions come later, if necessary at all. These deeper interventions, involving core person schemas and enduring beliefs, require time for the therapist to expand and revise earlier formulations.

Termination can then be considered, it is the topic of the next chapter. Discussions about the patient terminating treatment may occur before complete working through can be accomplished. In fact "complete working through" is an ideal, seldom a therapeutic reality. All people have a residue of conflicts, contradictory beliefs, and existential dilemmas that are difficult to confront.

The goal is for the patient to adequately work through his or her problems rather than arriving at a total resolution of conflicts. As will be discussed in the next chapter, the therapist can help the patient clarify the
personal issues that remain important and unresolved. The future can be
examined and confronted with plans; the patient can then continue a personal developmental course on his or her own. The patient can advance in
character strength through normal coping with problems and engaging in
existential struggles, and so progress along a course in life would otherwise
be disrupted and impaired by the presence of the stress response syndrome.

CHAPTER 7

Terminating Treatment

Upon arriving at a joint decision with the patient to end regularly scheduled treatment sessions, the therapist's aim is to help the patient work through emotions about separation and to reinforce adaptive new beliefs and attitudes. Termination of the treatment represents the ending of a valuable period of support and can threaten reenactment of the patient's sense of personal vulnerability during the recent stressor events. For this reason, therapists should introduce plans for the time of terminating treatment several sessions before the final one. The loss of the alliance can then be faced gradually, actively rather than passively, within a shared context.

It may be helpful to inform the patient that he or she will continue to process stress-inducing experiences after the conclusion of therapy sessions. Some emotional reactions that have subsided may recur. Their reappearance should not lead to dismay; it may be a part of normal recovery rather than a sign of relapse. For example, treatment may begin but not complete what will eventually be a satisfactory mourning process.

The establishment, by mutual agreement, of a rational end point may still be irrationally interpreted as a rejection. The patient may feel unworthy and/or believe that the therapist is reacting in retaliation to the patient's hostile ideas and feelings. When interpreting such transference reactions, the therapist can indicate whether and how such attitudes and reactions link to the stressor event; they can be considered as an opportunity for working on the event's implications. Equally important, the therapist can encourage the patient to discuss the meaning of the therapy experience, to share positive feelings, and to be able to say "thank you."

Although the following case example ends in termination, it first presents the case formulation and stages of therapy as a review of the issues presented in this book.

CASE EXAMPLE: CONNIE

Connie had completed college and was moving about in temporary employments. She was also frequently changing intimate attachments. Her life was suddenly shattered by the unexpected death of her father. Although her mother and siblings grieved, Connie was far more distraught. She was first seen in therapy 6 weeks after her father's death, at which time she was diagnosed as having a complicated grief disorder and a histrionic personality style.

Configurational Analysis

The following formulation for Connie is presented in the configurational analysis format of 1) phenomena, 2) states, 3) topics of concern and defensive control processes, and 4) identity and relationship concepts.

Phenomena to Explain

Since her father's unexpected death, Connie had been confused, felt intensely sad, and experienced a loss of initiative. She faltered badly in her career activities and felt that her intimate relationships had come unglued. Her sense of identity and her sense of having a future direction were more diffuse to her now than before the death.

States of Mind

Connie desired to feel composed and well connected to others; instead, she was often in a dreaded state, one of feeling flooded with grief and sadness. She feared that others would see her sobbing in a messy, out-of-control manner. She assumed a problematic compromise state of inertia in which she sat about, waiting for she knew not what. Entry into a protective compromise state allowed her to regain more of a sense of self-control. In this aloof, composed state, Connie seemed poised but felt inwardly estranged from any real contact with others; she was not spontaneous, had no sense of empathy, and was not intimate with anyone (Figure 7–1).

Topics of Concern and Defensive Control Processes

Connie's central concern was she could not find a consistent personal attitude of how she felt about her father and his death. She puzzled over

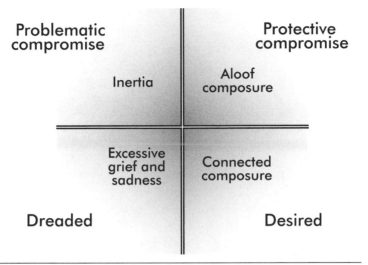

Problematic compromise	Protective compromise
Inertia	Aloof composure
Excessive grief and sadness	Connected composure
Dreaded	Desired

FIGURE 7–1. Configuration of states for Connie.

whether he had really loved her. He had ignored her concerns during the past 2 years, and she had intrusive memories of how she had not related well to him during that time. Her defensive response was to try not to think about it and to avoid conversing on the topic. When asked how she felt about seeing her father so infrequently in the last few years, she repeated, "I don't know." In addition to the father topic, she felt unresolved about an intimate relationship and was concerned about her lack of personal productivity.

Identity and Relationships

Connie presented an idealized positive relationship with her father, one of mutual prizing and of sharing intelligent and compassionate traits. In a desired relationship, she would be an intelligent woman prized by an equal companion or mentor. She warded off an alternative view in which she perceived herself as a disgusting, wailing waif, too weak to be like—or of interest to—her father or other "superior-type" men or women. She also felt angry, as if abandoned by an irresponsible caretaker. In this dreaded role relationship model, she pined, was deserted, and then reacted with anger, which had to be warded off out of fear that it might harm her irresponsible caretaker (Figure 7–2).

Connie protected herself with a facade of composure, as if insulated from potential critics, but she found this difficult to maintain because it felt

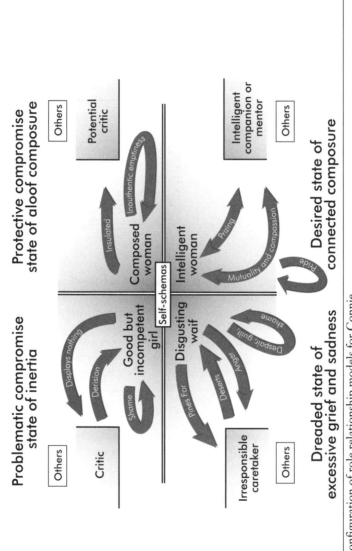

FIGURE 7–2.   Configuration of role relationship models for Connie.

inauthentic. She assumed a problematic compromise state in which she experienced herself as a good but incompetent girl who was ashamed because she was unproductive and, therefore, degraded by a superior critic.

Integration and Treatment Planning

Connie felt unable to go through a grieving process alone—such an experience would be too intense and confusing. The treatment plan involved facilitating Connie's mourning by establishing a safe time-limited relationship without fostering undue dependency. The aim was to explore how, and then why, she warded off certain topics about her father. With that process under way, the therapist believed that he could help Connie to integrate and harmonize contradictions in her memories and fantasies, thereby gaining a restored sense of self-efficacy; this, in turn, would affect her actions toward advancing her career and developing more adaptive social relationships. The first goal would be to reduce Connie's sense of confusion through providing clarity of focus and initial support.

Stages of Treatment

Initial Support

In the first two sessions, the therapist provided support by listening to Connie's story; after these sessions, she felt that she had regained control. She could allow herself to feel pangs of sadness without entering a flooded, overwhelmed, and out-of-control state. By the fourth session, Connie felt much less confused or anxious and experienced less intrusive and avoidant symptoms. She began to wonder if she were done in therapy and questioned whether more sessions would be worthwhile. It was natural for her to want to avoid the emotional turbulence of reviewing her relationship with her father.

Exploration of Meanings

In spite of Connie's reluctance, the therapist focused on the loss of her father and its meaning to her. Exploring this topic helped Connie to conceptualize and discuss how she sometimes felt either too weak or too revengeful toward her father. A view of herself as evil was activated by her reacting to his death as if she had wanted it; she dimly realized how intensely hostile she felt toward her father for his perceived betrayals. This became clearer as she described memories of how her father had scorned her and lied to her in recent years.

Connie also explored how she felt weak for not living up to her father's ideals and her regret that he had died before she could reestablish, as she hoped, the mutual relationship of admiration and respect that she had not experienced since their mutual idealization in her early teens. Her plan had been to convince him that her own modified career line and lifestyle would lead to many worthwhile accomplishments.

Improving Coping

The therapist pointed out to Connie that she sometimes reacted to him as if she expected his derision—as though she had an image of herself as bad and defective. She acknowledged that she also did this with her boyfriend. The therapist contrasted her expectation of shame with more realistic expectations of being treated by others as a worthwhile person. He suggested that she be alert to down talking herself and to counteract her lapses in esteem with more appropriate self-appraisals. The therapist also encouraged Connie to compare her feelings about losing her father to those about separating from her boyfriend and leaving the therapist when treatment was complete. Doing so would help her clarify and deal with the confusing mixture of sadness, humiliation, and rage that accompanied the idea of any separation.

Working Through

During childhood and early adolescence, Connie had viewed her father as strong and omnipotent. In late adolescence and early adulthood, however, she had seen his deceits. In a magical way, after his death, she evoked the earlier view of her father's omnipotence and perceived his death as a deliberate desertion of her. She felt that she deserved this separation because she was unworthy of his love. The therapist countered this theme with more realistic beliefs.

The next theme for repeated work was warded-off anger at her father. Connie believed that her hostility might have been magically harmful, as in a death wish. The therapist clarified and challenged this belief. The father and the daughter were human; Connie's father was not omnipotent, not always right or wrong, but mortal and in part flawed. His death was not an intentional desertion, nor had it occurred because she willed it to happen.

It was difficult for Connie to give up her magical idealization of her father, because she sometimes viewed herself as a person too weak to survive without a strong father. It was hard for her to confront her primitive feeling that she wanted revenge for his deceits, because no one, certainly not her introjected father, would love an angry person. This view was linked with memories involving her mother. Connie felt that her father did not love her mother because "Mother often cried and angrily railed at him." The therapist pointed out that Connie had wanted to be more like her father and unlike her mother. Now she would learn from her own convictions what she could become in the future. Efforts were made to help Connie accept the ambivalence in memories of both her father and mother and to consider her parents as having traits she both valued and disliked.

After her father's funeral, Connie had turned to her lover for consolation and sympathy. Connie, however, had selected a man who, like her father, was superior, cool, and remote. When she searched for her ideal of him as a strong, supportive figure, she found that he was unable to provide what she wanted. Moreover, he was repelled by her sorrow and dependency and abandoned her. Connie had to work through her grief for this loss of confidence in her boyfriend, the loss of her father, and the loss of her idealizing naivete. For her, the working-through stage of treatment involved issues about personality development.

Connie gradually became able to more frequently achieve a desired state of connected composure with the therapist. She expected to be able to work on forming less dependent and more mutual relationships after the conclusion of treatment. It was with much less frequency and intensity that she experienced the dreaded state of excessive grief and sadness (Figure 7–1). States of inertia also occurred with reduced frequency. Although Connie still entered a protective state of aloof composure when she felt threatened, she felt threatened less frequently by her own emotionality than she had before therapy. These changes were discussed and a time of termination was set for 1 month in the future (she was being seen once a week).

Terminating

The idea of termination was associated with the centrally important father-loss topic. The end of therapy threatened Connie with the loss of a relationship with a kind, sustaining figure like her idealized father. This theme continued the focus on mourning by actively facing rather than avoiding the issues of who Connie was, what she needed, and what she could tolerate. During this final stage of treatment, the focus was also on Connie's future plans. This process included bolstering her realistically competent, rather than her dependently weak, beliefs about her ability to become skillful and accomplished.

CONCLUSIONS

The stages of evaluation, support, exploring meanings, improving coping, working through, and termination coexist, although for didactic purposes they were discussed in sequential chapters. Formulation begins during evaluation, but it is revised and elaborated on from beginning to end. Termination is especially important in stress response syndromes because it constitutes a loss and thus symbolically relates to the loss components found in most stressor events. Even if the stressor event involved no physical changes to the self or changes in connections with others, the person usually emerges having lost a sense of personal invulnerability. It is for this reason that it is important to allude to termination in the early stages of treatment. Subsequently, during the final stage, a review of past, present, and future attitudes about loss can provide a context for considering what was achieved during treatment. The therapist may also discuss what will be gained by continuing the work of mourning after the conclusion of therapy. As with Connie, the goal is to approach such issues actively and rationally, rather than passively or with outdated beliefs.

CHAPTER 8

Assessment of Outcome

Assessment of the level of stress-specific symptoms over time can usefully accompany treatment. A patient self-report measure employed for this purpose is the Impact of Event Scale (IES; Horowitz et al. 1979), which appeared earlier in this volume (see Table 2–3 in Chapter 2). The patient or the therapist specifies the relevant stressor event (or series of events) at the top of the form. This specification provides a specific referent (or focus) for each individual patient. The patient then endorses any of the listed intrusive and avoidant experiences that have occurred within the past 7 days. The IES can be periodically readministered to track the patient's adaptation to the specific stressor. Comparison scores for this widely used scale were provided in Table 2–4 of Chapter 2 (Horowitz et al. 1993). The IES has excellent psychometric properties (Briere and Elliot 1998; Joseph 2000; Larsson 2000; Sundin and Horowitz 2002).

There are 15 items in each IES. Each item is rated by the patient on a 4-point scale consisting of "not at all," "rarely," "sometimes," and "often." To derive a sum of scores, these responses are weighted as follows:

- Not at all=0
- Rarely=1
- Sometimes=3
- Often=5

The IES contains two subscales: Intrusion and Avoidance. The Intrusion subscale score is derived by adding items 1, 4, 5, 6, 10, 11, and 14. The Avoidance subscale score is derived by adding items 2, 3, 7, 8, 9, 12, 13, and 15. An IES total is the sum of the Intrusion and Avoidance subscales. The cutoff points for the IES (Intrusion plus Avoidance subscale scores) are as follows:

- Low=below 8.5
- Medium=between 8.5 and 19.0
- High=19.0 or more

A score of *low* denotes symptoms of probable subclinical significance, *high* those of likely clinical significance, and *medium* those requiring further clinical judgment as to pathology.

Instruments such as the Positive States of Mind Scale (Adler et al. 1998; Horowitz et al. 1988; Table 8–1) can be used to quickly assess impairments in positive life activities, as can the Self-Regard Questionnaire (Horowitz et al. 1995; Table 8–2). The author holds the copyright for the scales shown in Tables 2–3, 8–1, and 8–2 and gives the reader permission to copy and use them in his or her own practice. Many other scales are available for assessment of posttraumatic stress disorder (PTSD), grief, rape trauma, stress symptoms, general symptoms, life functioning, and well-being (Breslau 1999a, 1999b; Foa et al. 2000). Compilations of these instruments are available in publications by the American Psychological Association (www.apa.org), the American Psychiatric Association (www.psych.org), and the International Society for Traumatic Stress Studies (www.istss.org).

EFFICACY OF PHARMACOTHERAPY

There are many studies of all types of treatment modalities and drugs for all types of stress response syndromes (Foa et al. 2000). Selecting from research available at this writing, I first review research findings of studies using selective serotonin reuptake inhibitor (SSRI) medications. In a 12-week double-blind study of acute PTSD treatment, Davidson et al. (2001a, 2001b) found that patients treated with sertraline had a significantly steeper improvement slope than did patients given a placebo. Adverse effects significantly more common in subjects taking sertraline compared with those on placebo included insomnia, diarrhea, nausea, fatigue, and decreased appetite. The study sample was recruited from a clinical population and also through the use of advertising.

Sertraline treatment was initiated at 25 mg/day with flexible daily dos-

TABLE 8–1. Positive States of Mind Scale

Instructions: Circle 0 to 3 for each type of experience according to your judgment about the past 7 days.

	Unable to have it	Trouble having it	Limited in having it	Have it well
1. **Focused attention:** Feeling able to work on a task you want or need to do, without many distractions from within yourself.	0	1	2	3
2. **Productivity:** Feeling of flow and satisfaction without severe frustrations, perhaps while doing something new to solve problems or to express yourself creatively.	0	1	2	3
3. **Responsible caretaking:** Feeling that you are doing what you should do to take care of yourself or someone else in a way that helps meet life's necessities.	0	1	2	3
4. **Restful repose:** Feeling relaxed, without distractions or excessive tension, without difficulty in stopping it when you want to.	0	1	2	3
5. **Sensuous pleasure:** Being able to enjoy bodily senses, enjoyable intellectual activity, doing things you ordinarily like, such as listening to music, enjoying the outdoors, lounging in a hot bath, being able to enjoy kissing, caressing, or intercourse.	0	1	2	3
6. **Sharing:** Being able to commune with others in an empathic, close way, perhaps with a feeling of joint purposes or values.	0	1	2	3

Scoring: Take the value circled as the score for each of the six items. The item scores can also all be added together as a single crude measure of functionality. Scores in the higher numerical range (15–18) are considered better than those in the lower ranges.

Source. Adler NE, Horowitz M, Garcia A, et al.: "Additional Validation of a Scale to Assess Positive States of Mind." *Psychosomatic Medicine* 60:26–32, 1998; Horowitz MJ, Adler N, Kegeles S: A Scale for Measuring the Occurrence of Positive States of Mind. *Psychosomatic Medicine* 50:477–483, 1988. Used with permission. Copyright M. Horowitz.

TABLE 8–2. Self-Regard Questionnaire

Instructions: Circle one number for each question below indicating your average over the past 7 days, including today.

Sense of my facial appearance

	1	2	3	4	5	6	7	8	9	10	
Least healthy I can really look											Most healthy I can really look

Sense of fatigue

	1	2	3	4	5	6	7	8	9	10	
Most tired I can really get											Least tired I can really get

Sense of healthy body

	1	2	3	4	5	6	7	8	9	10	
Least healthy my body can feel											Most healthy my body can feel

Sense of healthy mind

	1	2	3	4	5	6	7	8	9	10	
Least healthy my mind can feel											Most healthy my mind can feel

Sense of my identity as a whole person

	1	2	3	4	5	6	7	8	9	10	
Least clear sense of myself as a whole person											Most clear sense of myself as a whole person

Scoring: Take the total of five scores by adding each number circled. A high score (40–50) indicates high self-regard for the week and is better than low scores.

Source. Horowitz M, Sonneborn D, Sugahara C, et al.: Self-Regard: A New Measure. *American Journal of Psychiatry* 153:382–385, 1996. Used with permission. Copyright M. Horowitz.

ing thereafter in the range of 50–200 mg. The majority of precipitating traumatic events were physical or sexual assaults; the second most frequent event category was seeing someone hurt or killed. The manufacturer of the drug sertraline supported the study.

Davidson et al. (2001a, 2001b) also found sertraline to be effective in a continuation treatment study (a 24-week additional period), an open-label study, and a maintenance treatment study (a 28-week double-blind, placebo-controlled trial with patients who had previously responded to acute treatment). The maintenance study compared 46 patients on sertraline with 50 patients randomly assigned to a placebo. Patients who received placebo were more than 6 times as likely to experience relapse as were patients who received sertraline in the additional 7-month period of maintenance treatment. The average sertraline dosage at this end point was 137 mg/day.

In another report (Brady et al. 2000), about 200 patients were randomized to receive either sertraline (at an average dosage of 133 mg/day) or a placebo. In both groups, many subjects discontinued the treatment for a variety of reasons. In two patients, sertraline was discontinued because of laboratory abnormalities, one involving decreases in hemoglobin, and the other involving an increase in liver enzymes. Although both sertraline-treated and placebo-treated patients experienced a reduction in PTSD symptoms, a sharper rate of decrease was noted with sertraline. Depression symptoms also declined more sharply in the group that received the active medication. The authors of this study pointed out that the benefits of pharmacotherapy in the treatment of PTSD have been shown to be moderate and possibly lower than those of cognitive or behavioral therapies. Before receiving treatment, patients in this study had a mean symptom duration of 10 years. The types of trauma experienced ranged from physical or sexual assaults (in the majority of patients) to witnessing violence and miscellaneous other events such as kidnapping (Brady et al. 2000).

Other SSRI agents may soon be approved by the U.S. Food and Drug Administration for treatment of PTSD. Paroxetine, for example, was found to be effective in the treatment of chronic PTSD in a placebo-controlled study (Marshall et al. 2001). The subjects were male and female outpatients, ages 18 years or older, who met criteria for chronic PTSD. The fixed doses used were 20 and 40 mg/day of paroxetine. Patients receiving active medication demonstrated significantly greater improvement on primary outcome measures compared with placebo-treated patients. The most commonly reported adverse effects associated with paroxetine, with an incidence at least twice that of placebo, included diarrhea, abnormal ejaculation, impotence, nausea, insomnia, and somnolence. The manufacturer of the drug paroxetine supported this study.

EFFICACY OF PSYCHOTHERAPY

The type of integrated psychotherapy outlined in this book combines pharmacological, behavioral, cognitive, and psychodynamic principles. My colleagues and I assessed change in groups of patients examined before and after such treatments at a time when we used mainly a cognitive-psychodynamic integration. Measures included the IES (Horowitz et al. 1979; Zilberg et al. 1982); the Stress Response Rating Scale (clinician's assessment) (Horowitz 1976; Weiss et al. 1984); the Patterns of Individualized Change Scales (DeWitt et al. 1983; Kaltreider et al. 1981; Weiss et al. 1985), which assess work, intimacy, caretaking, and other life functions; and assessments of the therapeutic alliance (Marmar et al. 1987; Marziali et al. 1981), therapist actions (Hoyt 1980; Hoyt et al. 1981), and patients' motivations (Rosenbaum and Horowitz 1983). A dispositional measure of importance was the Organizational Level of Self and Other Schematization (Horowitz 1979, 1987, 1998; Horowitz et al. 1984a). A dispositional measure assesses some pretrauma aspect of personality, however, a pretrauma disposition is difficult to assess after the patient has developed a stress response syndrome.

Using these measures to study 52 patients who developed stress response syndromes after the death of a family member, we examined the results of 12-session, individual time-limited therapy (as reported in detail in Horowitz et al. 1984a). Before treatment, patients in our sample had symptom levels comparable to those of other psychiatric outpatient samples studied in treatment research: on the Symptom Checklist—90 (SCL-90; Derogatis et al. 1976), which measures general psychiatric symptoms rated by self-report, the mean symptom level at treatment onset for our sample was 1.19 (SD=0.59). This level is almost identical to the level of 1.25 (SD=0.39) reported by Derogatis et al. (1976) for a sample of 209 symptomatic psychiatric outpatients before treatment. In our study, the mean SCL-90 depression subscale score at intake was 1.81; in the Derogatis et al. study, it was 1.87. The scores for anxiety were also comparable: 1.39 in our sample and 1.49 in the sample of Derogatis et al.

A significant improvement was seen in all symptom outcome variables when pretherapy scores were compared with follow-up scores. Our results can be expressed in terms of the standardized, mean-difference, effect-size coefficient, as recommended by Cohen (1979) for pre- and posttreatment data. Cohen defined a large effect as 0.80 or greater. Our large effect sizes were in the domain of symptoms and ranged from 1.21 to 0.71. Changes in work, interpersonal functioning, and capacity for intimacy on the Patterns of Individualized Change Scales indicated improvements that were more moderate (Horowitz et al. 1986).

This cognitive-psychodynamic approach has been found to be effective in studies by other investigators in other institutions. A study conducted by Brom et al. (1989) in the Netherlands found this approach to be as effective as behavioral therapy in the treatment of PTSD. It was also as effective as cognitive-behavioral therapy in the treatment of major depressive disorders (Gallagher-Thompson et al. 1990; Thompson et al. 1987, 1991). In both of these studies, the therapy groups did better than the wait-list control groups. In a meta-analytic review of equivalent studies, this cognitive-psychodynamic approach was one of the treatments found to be effective (Crits-Christoph et al. 1988; see also Sherman 1998). The synthesis of cognitive with psychodynamic theory is described elsewhere (Horowitz 1998), as is the systematic method of formulation outlined in Chapter 2 (Horowitz 1997).

Cognitive-behavioral therapy without psychodynamic components is also an effective treatment (Foa et al. 2000). The various cognitive-behavioral therapies have lent themselves well to manuals specifying how treatment is to be conducted, to studies of therapists' compliance with manuals, and to brief approaches. As a result, many studies are available that demonstrate their effectiveness. A few representative studies are briefly reviewed below.

Early psychosocial treatment may help prevent a later need for medications or for treatment of a more chronic PTSD. In a study reported by Bryant and colleagues (1998), 24 participants with acute stress disorder following a civilian trauma were treated with either five sessions of cognitive-behavioral therapy or supportive counseling, usually within 2 weeks of their trauma. Six months after the trauma, there were fewer PTSD cases in the group that received cognitive-behavioral therapy (17%) than in the group that received the supportive counseling (67%). The group that received the cognitive-behavioral therapy had statistically significant reductions in intrusive thinking, avoidance, and depressive symptomatology in comparison with the other group. In this study, the cognitive-behavioral treatment consisted of education about trauma reactions, training in progressive muscle relaxation, imaginal exposure to traumatic memories, cognitive restructuring of fear-related beliefs, and graded in vivo exposure to avoided situations. In contrast, the supportive counseling program consisted of education about trauma and taught general problem-solving skills, with the therapist taking an unconditionally supportive role. Exposure and anxiety management techniques were specifically avoided.

Some treatments can be conducted in groups that focus on specific types of problems. For example, cognitive-behavioral therapy was effective in reducing insomnia and nightmare frequency in 62 participants who completed a 10-hour group treatment consisting of imagery rehearsal for nightmares and sleep hygiene, stimulus control, and sleep restriction for insomnia. The subjects were crime victims who subsequently developed PTSD (Krakow et al. 2001).

In instances of comorbidity, specific techniques for each problem can be combined. Brady et al. (2001) examined the effect of exposure therapy in 39 patients with concurrent PTSD and cocaine dependence. Imaginal and in vivo exposure therapy techniques were used to treat PTSD symptoms, and cognitive-behavioral techniques were used to curb cocaine usage. The dropout rate was high, with less than half of the sample completing at least 10 sessions. Such attrition is not uncommon in cohorts of substance- abusing persons. Those who did complete 10 or more sessions demonstrated significant reductions in both PTSD symptoms and cocaine use from baseline to the end of treatment.

Dismantling studies have also been conducted. Given that all psychotherapies have multiple components, the purpose of a dismantling study is to test a specific hypothetically important component to see if it is effective. For example, one such study examined eye movement desensitization and reprocessing (EMDR) to determine the specific effects of eye movement control by a therapist. Previous studies had shown that use of a treatment employing therapist control of eye movements reduced anxiety associated with visual traumatic memories (Shapiro 1989; Wilson et al. 1995). The investigators compared EMDR (Shapiro 1989) with all its components with EMDR minus the eye movement component. Both groups of patients showed similar levels of symptom reduction after treatment (Pitman et al. 1996). These results suggested to the investigators that exposure and/or other nonspecific therapy factors in the set of procedures were more critical for the therapy gains than the eye movement control itself.

The research discussed here represents just a few of the studies demonstrating the effectiveness of a variety of approaches to treatment of stress response syndromes. A more extensive literature goes beyond studies of PTSD and acute stress disorder to address other disorders precipitated by serious stressor events. This literature is rapidly changing. For therapists to keep current, Web sites may be helpful in addition to books and scientific journals. The National Center for PTSD (www.ncptsd.org), the International Society for Traumatic Stress Studies (www.istss.org), and MEDLINE are locations where new studies may be listed.

The studies published in journals tend to use a homogeneous patient group, usually homogeneous by diagnosis of PTSD. In actual clinical fact, such groups are heterogeneous even when they have a stressor event in common. Personality variation and prior trauma variation can make a difference. The studies also tend to use specific kinds of therapy (e.g., just behavioral, just cognitive, just brief dynamic psychotherapy, or just pharmacological management) rather than a clinician-based therapy in which individual choices of technique from a wide repertoire are selected and various specific methods are integrated. It is likely that a clinician with a wide repertoire of knowledge and with skills in case formulation could construct an individually tailored treatment that would achieve even higher levels of efficacy than those noted in formal research studies.

CONCLUSIONS

The main symptoms of stress response syndromes include a variety of intrusive and denial-numbing type deflections from a patient's normal conscious equilibrium. In addition, the patient experiences bodily disturbances, sleep changes, impairments in achieving ordinarily positive states of mind, and a diminished sense of having a coherent identity as well as experiencing infrequent feelings of good self-regard. These symptoms can be assessed with a variety of self-report scales and observer rating scales. By examining the measures over time, a clinician can tract changes during and after treatment. That is, by assessing the last week on a specific scale, both patient and clinician can learn if improvement is taking place over months or years.

Self-report and observer ratings, or diagnostic judgments, were taken by clinical investigators before, during, and after treatment in comparative trials. Often the inclusion and exclusion criteria, length of treatment, the actions of the therapist, and the single medication used were tightly controlled in the design of these formal research studies. Many used manuals defining therapist actions and therapists were assessed for adherence to the manual. These design factors do not apply to the clinching treating individuals who are not in a research study. For the clinician in practice, a case specific choice of how to integrate treatments has been suggested. Of course the clinician should keep abreast of research on the efficacy of various approaches and be alert to the yet to be discovered techniques for facilitating change.

CHAPTER 9

A Few Caveats

Some underdeveloped areas of this book include posttraumatic stress disorder (PTSD) in Vietnam veterans, group treatment, treatment of the effects of early childhood trauma in adult patients, torture, and terrorism. Brief comments on each of these topics follow.

POSTTRAUMATIC STRESS DISORDER IN VIETNAM VETERANS

In the years immediately following the Vietnam War, for various reasons, there was an underrepresentation of stress response syndromes in Veterans Administration Medical Centers (Horowitz and Solomon 1975; Shepard 2001). Systematic clinical research has subsequently documented a high frequency of PTSD in combat-exposed military personnel (Kulka et al. 1990). Many in this population still need treatment, and some have very complex problems. For veterans with the most serious and difficult cases, even long-term, intensive inpatient treatment has not achieved a high cure rate, although one study found that such treatment did improve morale and reduce violent episodes (Johnson et al. 1996).

THERAPIST-LED AND MUTUAL-HELP THERAPY GROUPS

I believe that many of the principles described in this volume can also be used in therapist-led groups. Although I have underemphasized group approaches because my own clinical research has focused on individualized approaches, I encourage the reader to seek more information in that realm. Mutual-help groups are also likely to be beneficial (Lieberman 2001; Lieberman et al. 1973; Marmar et al. 1988).

CHILDHOOD TRAUMA AFFECTING ADULT PATIENTS

A great deal has been written about childhood incest and abuse, repressed memories, and adult effects (e.g., Herman 1992). I have not covered such topics systematically here. For patients with predominately chronic adult personality problems to which childhood traumas contributed, the guidelines offered in this book may not be exactly on target. I have focused on adult stressor events that may activate memories of childhood traumas but not on extensive work to repair chronic personality damage from early trauma.

TRANSGENERATIONAL TRAUMA

Images of horror are transmitted by story repetition, and some kinds of reactivity are communicated nonverbally. In genocidal disasters, the terror inflicted on those fortunate enough to survive can potentially be passed on to their children who come to believe that terrible things will happen to them in the future (Danieli 1998). The transmitted images of horror become schemas of expectation that can drain hope and disrupt equilibrium even in grandchildren. In some instances, a role reversal occurs and themes of revenge are passed on. Both fear and revenge preoccupations can reach pathological proportions.

Beyond images of horror, transgenerational communication of coping and defensive stances may occur. Parents with stress-induced regulatory failures can have extreme emotional lability. Their children may not learn adequate skills to self-regulate their own emotion. In addition, feelings of shame about uncontrolled expressions of intense emotion, stigmatization as a victim, and guilt about having survived may be passed on. Inchoate and implicit ideas like these can be made lucid and explicit in treatment if the therapy is conducted in a very supportive and time-extended manner. Long-term, developmentally oriented approaches have not been fully explored in this book.

TORTURE

Victims of torture may have special problems in resolving their stress response syndromes. In addition to the physical injury, handicaps, terrible memories, and other sequelae, they have been dehumanized and forced into extreme helplessness (Elsass 1997). At times they have been coerced to betray others; at other times, they have been sadistically used as toys for evil excitement. This extreme break in connection to a shared human condition has been likened to a murder of the soul, a torment beyond the direct effects of an extraordinarily severe set of life events. Some kind of spiritual restoration may need to be added to treatment plans.

TERRORISM

As I conclude the writing of this manuscript, we are 3 months into a war on terrorism initiated by the September 11, 2001, devastation of the World Trade Center in New York City and the Pentagon in Washington, D.C. Planes loaded with jet fuel, passengers, crew, and suicidal hijackers were flown into buildings that subsequently collapsed, killing thousands. Some survivors and many friends and relatives have already manifested a variety of stress syndromes. A proportion of those fighting in a war on terrorism will also have stress response syndromes. People in New York and elsewhere have developed conditioned fear responses to certain locations. Although this book has addressed treatment of such conditions, it has not discussed specifically the spread of terror to those who witness these events on television.

Phobias and generalized anxiety as well as a variety of adjustment problems may affect hundreds of thousands of members of an involved population who participate via the media and through their future expectations. This spreading impact is the aim of terrorists. In the ripples of fear after a terrorist attack, the public health goal is a reduction of irrational and disabling levels of fright and/or rage. Preventive interventions can emphasize realistic preparedness and ways to 1) reduce irrational exaggerations of personal risks, 2) foster a feeling of being connected to others, and 3) increase a sense of being engaged in active coping. Public media should provide accurate information (rather than blanket denials of threat), communicate the expectation of a gradual habituation to the realistic threat (rather than the anticipation of fright forever), and offer practical information on appropriate responses to various future eventualities (rather than fostering passive fear).

CONCLUSIONS

Intrusions and avoidances are deflections from well-modulated conscious experiences. Both stem from changes in emotional appraisals of the world and alterations in the functioning of cognitive regulatory processes. Intrusions interrupt the focus of volitional attention and occur in spite of inhibitory efforts. Avoidances are the product of defensive aims to stifle otherwise expectable emotions. Intrusions can be both adaptive (initiating information processing) and maladaptive (producing symptoms). Avoidances can be both adaptive (promoting equilibrium) and maladaptive (reducing information processing).

Attenuation of intrusions and avoidances occurs with desensitization of conditioned associations and assimilation of meanings of the stressor event into the person's preexisting schematic structure. This process leads to a reduction in emotional alarm reactions from recollection of traumatic events or confrontation of trigger stimuli. Having fewer alarm reactions makes high levels of control less necessary. With information processing less stifled by controls, schemas of self and other can be updated to accord with new realities.

Accommodation to new realities includes review of traumatic memories. The process is not entirely under conscious control. A shift from denial into intrusive recollection might take place just when a person thinks that his or her stress is over. Transition into remembrance and emotion may occur only after the person feels relatively safe. Such increased recollections of stressor events with feelings of increased safety from harm suggest shifts have occurred in nonconscious processes of control. Preconscious appraisals say, in effect, "now is an acceptable time to assess this memory." Of course, transitions from numb states to emotional states also occur with triggers that prime warded-off mental contents and with stimuli that evoke conditioned fear responses.

Good treatment affects both controls and the emotional–ideational processing that is regulated. The therapist is dealing with the patient's conscious thought and is also influencing the patient's preconscious processing and unconscious storage of knowledge (realistic and unrealistic). Various psychological, biological, and social interventions may influence the patient's controls, emotionality, and information-processing capacity. These matters are complex; individual case formulation and treatment planning is advocated.

Because mastery of stressors involves both conscious and unconscious mental processing, and because the stressed person is on overload, integration of stressor memories into schemas is not rapid and seamlessly progressive. The individual continues to experience states of mind in which memories are processed differently. For example, when a patient is making a conscious effort to recall a stressful event, his or her memory might become accessible, inaccessible, then accessible again.

As stress is experienced and then mastered, the person's identity and affiliative relationships change. Optimum treatment fosters a self-developmental process. Although some losses can never be compensated, the person may still gain new areas of strength.

Some stress response syndromes are chronic and recurrent. The stronger the individual can become with help, the better he or she will be able to counteract long-term problems. Even chronic problems can be attenuated with reductions in substance abuse, anxiety, depression, anomie, poverty, ignorance, and impoverished coping skills. Trauma can have terrible and long-lasting effects, but stress response syndromes are very treatable, and an evaluation of them in a context of hope begins that effort.

References

Adler NE, Horowitz M, Garcia A, et al: Additional validation of a scale to assess positive states of mind. Psychosom Med 60:26–32, 1998

Allen JG: Coping With Trauma: A Guide to Self-Understanding. Washington, DC, American Psychiatric Press, 1999

American Psychiatric Association: Diagnostic and Statistical Manual of Mental Disorders, 4th Edition. Washington, DC, American Psychiatric Association, 1994

Amick-McMullan A, Kilpatrick DG, Veronen LJ, et al: Family survivors of homicide victims: theoretical perspectives and an exploratory study. J Trauma Stress 2:21–35, 1989

Andrews B, Brewin CR, Ochera J, et al: Characteristics, context and consequences of memory recovery among adults in therapy. Br J Psychiatry 175:141–146, 1999

Bandura A: Self-efficacy: toward a unified theory of behavioral change. Psychol Rev 84:191–215, 1977

Basch M: Doing Psychotherapy. New York, Basic Books, 1980

Beck A: Cognitive Therapy and Emotional Disorders. New York, International Universities Press, 1976

Benzer D, Smith D, Miller N: Detoxification from benzodiazepine use: strategies and schedules for clinical practice. Psychiatric Annals 25:180–185, 1995

Brady K, Pearlstein T, Asnis GM, et al: Efficacy and safety of sertraline treatment of posttraumatic stress disorder: a randomized controlled trial. JAMA 283: 1837–1844, 2000

Brady KT, Dansky BS, Back SE, et al: Exposure therapy in the treatment of PTSD among cocaine-dependent individuals: preliminary findings. J Subst Abuse Treat 21:47–54, 2001

Bramsen I, Dirkzwager AJE, van der Ploeg HM: Predeployment personality traits and exposure to trauma as predictors of posttraumatic stress symptoms: a prospective study of former peacekeepers. Am J Psychiatry 157:1115–1119, 2000

Breslau N, Chilcoat HD, Kessler RC, et al: Previous exposure to trauma and PTSD effects of subsequent trauma: results from the Detroit area survey of trauma. Am J Psychiatry 156:902–907, 1999a

Breslau N, Peterson EL, Kessler RC, et al: Short screening scale for DSM-IV posttraumatic stress disorder. Am J Psychiatry 156:908–911, 1999b

Briere J, Elliott DM: Clinical utility of the Impact of Event Scale: psychometrics in the general population. Assessment 5:171–180, 1998

Brom D, Kleber RJ, Defares PB: Brief psychotherapy for traumatic stress disorders. J Consult Clin Psychol 57:607–612, 1989

Bryant RA: Cognitive behavioral therapy of violence-related posttraumatic stress disorder. Aggression and Violent Behavior 5:79–97, 2000

Bryant RA, Harvey AG, Dang ST, et al: Treatment of acute stress disorder: a comparison of cognitive-behavioral therapy and supportive counseling. J Consult Clin Psychol 66:862–866, 1998

Caplan G: An Approach to Community Mental Health. New York, Grune & Stratton, 1961

Card JJ: Epidemiology of PTSD in a national cohort of Vietnam veterans. J Clin Psychol 43:6–17, 1987

Chemtob CM, Hamada RS, Roitblat HL, et al: Anger, anger control, and impulsivity in combat-related post-traumatic stress disorder. J Consult Clin Psychol 62:827–832, 1994

Cohen J: Power Analyses for the Social and Behavioral Sciences. New York, Academic Press, 1979

Crits-Christoph P, Luborsky L, Dahl L, et al: Clinicians can agree in assessing relationship patterns in psychotherapy: the core conflictual relationship theme method. Arch Gen Psychiatry 45:1001–1004, 1988

Danieli Y: International Handbook of Multigenerational Legacies of Trauma. New York, Plenum, 1998

Davidson J[R], Pearlstein T, Londborg P, et al: Efficacy of sertraline in preventing relapse of posttraumatic stress disorder: results of a 28-week double-blind, placebo-controlled study. Am J Psychiatry 158:1974–1981, 2001a

Davidson JR, Rothbaum BO, van der Kolk BA, et al: Multicenter, double-blind comparison of sertraline and placebo in the treatment of posttraumatic stress disorder. Arch Gen Psychiatry 58:485–492, 2001b

Derogatis LR, Rickels K, Rock A: The SCL-90 and the MMPI: a step in the validation of a new self-report scale. Br J Psychiatry 128:280–289, 1976

DeWitt KN, Kaltreider NB, Weiss DS, et al: Judging change in psychotherapy: reliability of clinical formulations. Arch Gen Psychiatry 40:1121–1128, 1983

Elliott DM: Traumatic events: prevalence and delayed recall in the general population. J Consult Clin Psychol 65:811–820, 1997

Elsass P: Treating Victims of Torture and Violence. New York, New York University Press, 1997

Foa EB, Hearst-Ikeda D: Emotional dissociation in response to trauma, in Handbook of Dissociation. Edited by Michelson LK, Ray W. New York, Plenum, 1996, pp 207–224

Foa EB, Kozak MJ: Emotional processing of fear: exposure to corrective information. Psychol Bull 99:20–35, 1988

Foa EB, Meadows EA: Psychosocial treatments for posttraumatic stress disorder: a critical review. Annu Rev Psychol 48:449–480, 1997

Foa EB, Rothbaum BO: Treating the Trauma of Rape: Cognitive Behavioral Therapy for PTSD. New York, Guilford, 1998

Foa EB, Keane TM, Friedman MJ (eds): Effective Treatments for PTSD: Practice Guidelines From the International Society for Traumatic Stress Studies. New York, Guilford, 2000

Follette VM, Ruzek JI, Abueg FR: Cognitive-Behavioral Therapies for Trauma. New York, Guilford, 1993

Foreman C: Sun Valley disaster study (unpublished manuscript). Martinez, CA, Contra Costa Health Services, 1988

Frank JB, Kosten TR, Giller EL, et al: A randomized clinical trial of phenelzine and imipramine for posttraumatic stress disorder. Am J Psychiatry 145:1289–1291, 1988

Gallagher-Thompson P, Hanley-Peterson P, Thompson LW: Maintenance of gain versus relapse following brief therapy for depression. J Consult Clin Psychol 58:371–374, 1990

Geracioti TD, Baker DG, Ekhator NN, et al: CSF norepinephrine concentrations in posttraumatic stress disorder. Am J Psychiatry 158:1227–1230, 2001

Hammen C, Davila J, Brown G, et al: Psychiatric history and stress: predictors of severity of unipolar depression. J Abnorm Psychol 101:45–52, 1992

Harvey AG, Bryant RA: Dissociative symptoms in acute stress disorder. J Trauma Stress 12:673–680, 1999

Herman J: Trauma and Recovery. New York, Basic Books, 1992

Horowitz MJ: Stress Response Syndromes. Northvale, NJ, 1st Edition. Northvale, NJ, Jason Aronson, 1976

Horowitz MJ: Depressive disorders in response to loss, in Stress and Anxiety. Edited by Sarason IG, Spielberger CD. New York, Hemisphere, 1979, pp 235–255

Horowitz MJ: States of Mind, 2nd Edition. New York, Plenum, 1987

Horowitz MJ: Formulation as a Basis for Planning Psychotherapy. Washington, DC, American Psychiatric Press, 1997

Horowitz MJ: Cognitive Psychodynamics: From Conflict to Character. New York, Wiley, 1998

Horowitz MJ: Essential Papers on Posttraumatic Stress Disorders. New York, New York University Press, 1999

Horowitz MJ: Stress Response Syndromes. Northvale, NJ, 4th Edition. Northvale, NJ, Jason Aronson, 2001

Horowitz MJ, Solomon G: A prediction of stress response syndromes in Vietnam veterans. Journal of Social Issues 31:67–80, 1975

Horowitz MJ, Wilner N, Alvarez W: The Impact of Event Scale: a measure of subjective stress. Psychosom Med 41:209–218, 1979

Horowitz MJ, Wilner N, Kaltreider N, et al: Signs and symptoms of posttraumatic stress disorder. Arch Gen Psychiatry 37 (1):85–92, 1980

Horowitz MJ, Marmar C, Weiss DS, et al: Brief psychotherapy of bereavement reactions: the relationship of process to outcome. Arch Gen Psychiatry 41:438–448, 1984a

Horowitz MJ, Weiss DS, Kaltreider NB, et al: Reactions to death of a parent: results from patients and field subjects. J Nerv Ment Dis 172:383–392, 1984b

Horowitz MJ, Marmar C, Weiss D, et al: Comprehensive analysis of change after brief dynamic psychotherapy. Am J Psychiatry 143 (5):582–589, 1986

Horowitz MJ, Adler N, Kegeles S: A scale for measuring the occurrence of positive states of mind. Psychosom Med 50:477–483, 1988

Horowitz MJ, Field N, Classen C: Stress response syndromes and their treatment, in Handbook of Stress: Theoretical and Clinical Aspects, 2nd Edition. Edited by Goldberger L, Breznitz S. New York, Free Press, 1993, pp 757–773

Horowitz M, Sonneborn D, Sugahara C, et al: Self-regard: a new measure. Am J Psychiatry 153:382–385, 1996

Horowitz MJ, Siegel B, Holen A, et al: Diagnostic criteria for complicated grief disorder. Am J Psychiatry 154:904–910, 1997

Hoyt M: Therapist and patient actions in "good" psychotherapy sessions. Arch Gen Psychiatry 37:159–161, 1980

Hoyt M, Marmar C, Horowitz MJ, et al: The Therapist Action Scale and the Patient Action Scale: instruments for the assessment of activities during dynamic psychotherapy. Psychotherapy: Theory, Research, and Practice 18:109–116, 1981

Jacobs SC: Traumatic Grief: Diagnosis, Treatment, Prevention. Philadelphia, PA, Bruner-Mazel, 1999

Jacobsen LK, Southwick SM, Kosten TR: Substance use disorders in patients with posttraumatic stress disorder: a review of the literature. Am J Psychiatry 158:1184–1190, 2001

Johnson D, Rosendreck R, Fontana A, et al: Outcome of intensive inpatient treatment for combat-related PTSD. Am J Psychiatry 153:771–777, 1996

Joseph S: Psychometric evaluation of Horowitz's Impact of Event Scale: a review. J Trauma Stress 13:101–113, 2000

Kaltreider NB, DeWitt K, Weiss D, et al: Patterns of individualized change scales. Arch Gen Psychiatry 38:1263–1269, 1981

Kardiner A, Spiegel H: War, Stress and Neurotic Illness. New York, P Hoeber, 1947

Kendler KS, Karkowski LM, Prescott CA: Causal relationship between stressful life events and the onset of major depression. Am J Psychiatry 156:837–841, 1999

Kessler RC, Sonnega A, Bromet E, et al: Posttraumatic stress disorder in the national comorbidity survey. Arch Gen Psychiatry 52:1048–1060, 1995

Kilpatrick DG, Veronen LJ: Treatment of Fear and Anxiety in Victims of Rape. Rockville, MD, National Institute of Mental Health, 1984

Kleber RJ, Figley CR, Gersons BPR (eds): Beyond Trauma, Cultural and Societal Dynamics. New York, Plenum, 1995

Klerman G, Weissman M (eds): New Applications of Interpersonal Psychotherapy. Washington, DC, American Psychiatric Press, 1993

Krakow B, Johnston L, Melendrez D, et al: An open-label trial of evidence-based cognitive behavior therapy for nightmares and insomnia in crime victims with PTSD. Am J Psychiatry 158:2043–2047, 2001

Kulka R, Schlenger W, Fairbank J, et al: Trauma and the Vietnam War Generation. New York, Brunner-Mazel, 1990

Ladwig KH, Schoefinius A, Dammann G, et al: Long-acting psychotraumatic properties of a cardiac arrest experience. Am J Psychiatry 156:912–919, 1999

Larsson G: Dimensional analysis of the Impact of Event Scale using structural equation modeling. J Trauma Stress 13:193–204, 2000

Laube J: Kalamata earthquake 1986: psychological reactions and a look at health care workers (unpublished manuscript). Hattiesburg, MI, University of Southern Mississippi School of Nursing, 1986

LeDoux JE: The Emotional Brain. New York, Simon & Schuster, 1996

LeDoux JE, Gorman JM: A call to action: overcoming anxiety through active coping. Am J Psychiatry 158:1953–1955, 2001

Lieberman MA, Golant M: Effectiveness of electronic support groups for women with breast cancer. Paper presented at American Psychological Association annual meeting, San Francisco, CA, October 3, 2001

Lieberman MA, Yalom ID, Miles MB: Encounter Groups: First Facts. New York, Basic Books, 1973

Lindemann E: Symptomatology and management of acute grief. Am J Psychiatry 101:141–148, 1944

Luborsky L: Principles of Psychoanalytic Psychotherapy: A Manual for Supportive Expressive Treatment. New York, Basic Books, 1984

Malan DH: Individual Psychotherapy and the Science of Psychodynamics. London, Butterworth, 1979

Mann J: Time-Limited Psychotherapy. Cambridge, MA, Harvard University Press, 1973

Marks I, Lovell K, Noshirvani H, et al: Treatment of posttraumatic stress disorder by exposure and/or cognitive restructuring: a controlled study. Arch Gen Psychiatry 55 (4):317–325, 1998

Marmar C, Marziali E, Horowitz MJ, et al: The development of the therapeutic alliance rating system, in Research in Psychotherapy. Edited by Greenberg L, Pinsoff W. New York, Guilford, 1987, pp 367–390

Marmar C, Horowitz MJ, Weiss D, et al: A controlled trial of brief psychotherapy and mutual help group treatment of conjugal bereavement. Am J Psychiatry 145:203–209, 1988

Marshall RD, Spitzer R, Liebowitz MR: Review and critique of the new DSM-IV diagnosis of acute stress disorder. Am J Psychiatry 156 (11):1677–1685, 1999

Marshall RD, Beebe KL, Oldham M, et al: Efficacy and safety of paroxetine treatment for chronic PTSD: a fixed-dose, placebo-controlled study. Am J Psychiatry 158:1982–1988, 2001

Marziali E, Marmar C, Krupnick J: Therapeutic alliance scales: development and relationship to therapeutic outcome. Am J Psychiatry 138, 361–364, 1981

Maskin M: Psychodynamic aspects of the war neuroses. Psychiatry 4:97–115, 1941

McFarlane AC: The longitudinal course of posttraumatic morbidity: the range of outcomes and their predictors. J Nerv Ment Dis 176:30–39, 1988

Meichenbaum D: Cognitive Behavior Modification: An Integrative Approach. New York, Plenum, 1977

Miller N: Benzodiazepine use in clinical practice: suggestions for prevention. American Journal of Preventive Psychiatry and Neurology 2:16–22, 1990

Parad H, Resnik H, Parad L: Emergency Mental Health Services and Disaster Management. New York, Prentice-Hall, 1976

Pitman RK, Orr SP, Altman B, et al: Emotional processing during eye movement desensitization and reprocessing therapy of Vietnam veterans with chronic posttraumatic stress disorder. Compr Psychiatry 37:419–429, 1996

Prigerson HG, Frank E, Kasl SV, et al: Complicated grief and bereavement-related depression as distinct disorders: preliminary empirical validation in elderly bereaved spouses. Am J Psychiatry 152 (1):22–30, 1995

Reynolds M, Brewin CR: Intrusive memories in depression and posttraumatic stress disorder. Behav Res Ther 37 (3):201–215, 1999

Rosenbaum R, Horowitz MJ: Motivation for psychotherapy: a factorial and conceptual analysis. Psychotherapy: Theory, Research, and Practice 20:346–354, 1983

Rosenbloom D, Williams MB: Life After Trauma: A Workbook for Healing. New York, Guilford, 1999

Schiralde GR: The Posttraumatic Stress Disorders Sourcebook. New York, Contemporary Books, 2000

Shapiro F: Efficacy of the eye movement desensitization procedure in the treatment of traumatic memories. Journal of Traumatic Stress 2:199–223, 1989

Shephard B: A War of Nerves: Soldiers and Psychiatrists in the Twentieth Century. Cambridge, MA, Harvard University Press, 2001

Sherman JJ: Effects of psychotherapeutic treatments for PTSD: a meta-analysis of controlled clinical trials. J Trauma Stress 11:413–435, 1998

Sifneos PE: Short-Term Psychotherapy and Emotional Crisis. Cambridge, MA, Harvard University Press, 1972

Solomon Z: Psychological sequelae of war: a 3-year prospective study of Israeli combat stress reaction casualties. J Nerv Ment Dis 177:342–346, 1989

Southwick SM, Krystal JH, Morgan CA, et al: Abnormal noradrenergic function in posttraumatic stress disorder. Arch Gen Psychiatry 50:266–274, 1993

Spiegel D: Trauma, dissociation, and memory. Ann N Y Acad Sci 821:225–237, 1997

Spiegel D, Classen C: Acute stress disorder, in Treatments of Psychiatric Disorders, 2nd Edition. Edited by Gabbard GO. Washington, DC, American Psychiatric Press, 1995, pp 1521–1535

Stein MB, Walker JR, Hazen AL, et al: Full and partial posttraumatic stress disorder: findings from a community survey. Am J Psychiatry 154:1114–1119, 1997

Steinglass P, Gerrity E: Natural disasters and post-traumatic stress disorder: short-term versus long-term recovery in two disaster-affected communities. J Appl Soc Psychol 20:1746–1765, 1990

Strupp HH, Binder JL: Psychotherapy in a New Key: A Guide to Time-Limited Dynamic Psychotherapy. New York, Basic Books, 1984

Sundin EC, Horowitz MJ: Impact of Event Scale: psychometric properties. Br J Psychiatry 180:205–209, 2002

Thompson LW, Gallagher D, Breckenridge JS: Comparative effectiveness of psychotherapies for depressed elders. J Geriatr Psychiatry 21:133–146, 1987

Thompson L, Gallagher-Thompson D, Fullerman A, et al: The effects of late-life spousal bereavement over a 30-month interval. Psychology and Aging 6 (3): 434–441, 1991

Trimble MR: Posttraumatic Neuroses. New York, Wiley, 1981

Wachtel PL: Psychoanalysis and Behavior Therapy: Toward an Integration. New York, Basic Books, 1977

Weiss DS, Horowitz MJ, Wilner N: Stress response rating scale: a clinician's measure. Br J Clin Psychol 23:202–215, 1984

Weiss D, DeWitt K, Kaltreider N, et al: A proposed method for measuring change beyond symptoms. Arch Gen Psychiatry 42:703–708, 1985

Williams LM, Banyard VL: Trauma and Memory. Thousand Oaks, CA, Sage, 1999

Wilson J, Lindy J: Countertransference in the Treatment of PTSD. New York, Guilford, 1994

Wilson JP, Raphael B (eds): International Handbook of Traumatic Stress Syndromes. New York, Plenum, 1993

Wilson SA, Becker LA, Tinker RH: Eye movement desensitization and reprocessing (EMDR) treatment for psychologically traumatized individuals. J Consult Clin Psychol 63:928–937, 1995

Yehuda R: Biology of posttraumatic stress disorder. J Clin Psychiatry 62 (suppl 17):41–46, 2001

Yehuda R, McFarlane AC: Conflict between current knowledge about posttraumatic stress disorder and its original conceptual basis. Am J Psychiatry 152:12, 1705–1713, 1995

Zatzick DF, Marmar CR, Weiss DS, et al: Does trauma-linked dissociation vary across ethnic groups? J Nerv Ment Dis 192:576–582, 1994

Zilberg N, Weiss D, Horowitz MJ: Impact of Event Scale: a cross-validation study and some empirical evidence. J Consult Clin Psychol 50:407–441, 1982

Index

Page numbers printed in **boldface** type refer to tables or figures.